Dementia
in the Family

Dementia
in the Family
Practical Advice from a Caregiver

Lee Cardwell

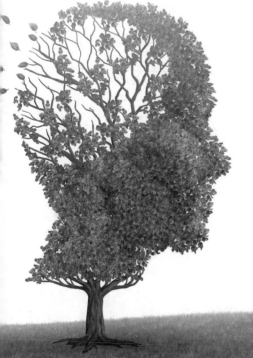

Self-Counsel Press
(a division of)
International Self-Counsel Press Ltd.
USA   Canada

Self-Counsel Press acknowledges the financial support of the Government of Canada through the Canada Book Fund (CBF) for our publishing activities.

Printed in Canada.

First edition: 2017

Library and Archives Canada Cataloguing in Publication

Cardwell, Lee, author
      Dementia in the family : practical advice from a caregiver / Lee Cardwell.

(Eldercare series)

Issued in print and electronic formats.
ISBN 978-1-77040-287-4 (softcover).—ISBN 978-1-77040-478-6 (EPUB).—ISBN 978-1-77040-479-3 (Kindle)
      1. Dementia.   2. Dementia—Patients--Family relationships.   I. Title.
II. Series: Eldercare series

RC521.C28 2017   616.8'31   C2017-900980-X
                                                              C2017-901070-0

Every effort has been made to obtain permission for quoted material. If there is an omission or error, the author and publisher would be grateful to be so informed. Excerpts from the following organizations and publications used with permission:

   Reproduced from Alzheimer's Association of Canada, "Know the 10 Warning Signs of Alzheimer's," http://www.alzheimer.ca/~/media/Files/national/AW2015/10WarningSigns_colour.pdf

   Reproduced from Alzheimers Association of Canada, "Alzheimers and Dementia," http://www.alz.org/dementia/types-of-dementia.asp#vascular

   Reproduced from B. Reisberg, S. H. Ferris, M. J. de Leon, and T. Crook, "The Global Deterioration Scale for Assessment of Primary Degenerative Dementia," *American Journal of Psychiatry* 139 (1982): 1136-1139.

Self-Counsel Press
(a division of)
International Self-Counsel Press Ltd.

Bellingham, WA   North Vancouver, BC
USA   Canada

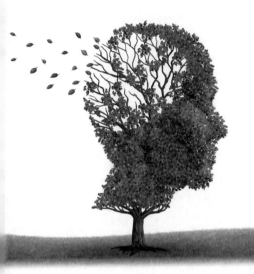

Contents

Notice to Readers

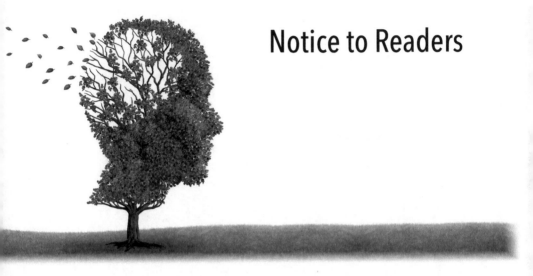

Laws are constantly changing. Every effort is made to keep this publication as current as possible. However, the author, the publisher, and the vendor of this book make no representations or warranties regarding the outcome or the use to which the information in this book is put and are not assuming any liability for any claims, losses, or damages arising out of the use of this book. The reader should not rely on the author or the publisher of this book for any professional advice. Please be sure that you have the most recent edition.

Dedication

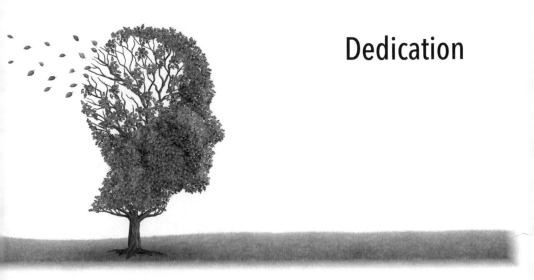

*I dedicate this book to the memory of my mother,
Shirley Hutchings, whom I still miss every day.*

Introduction

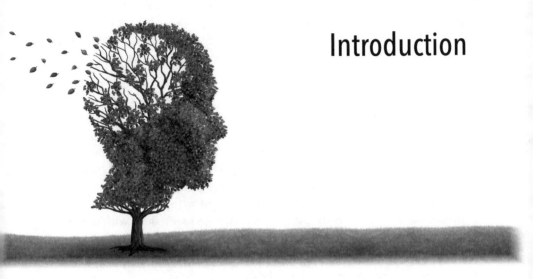

When you love someone, they never get lost; wherever they go, they are still somewhere in your heart and as long as they know that, they will always know that when they find you, they find themselves once again.

— Philippos

A vicious, uncaring thief is among us, and it is stealing the thoughts and memories of your family members and acquaintances. I have had to confront this villain over and over throughout the past several years. Many of us will have to tangle with this monster sometime, either for ourselves or for someone close to us. The thief has many names, but the one most common is "dementia."

Dementia comes from the Latin *de* ("without") and *mentia* ("mind") so it literally describes a state in which you are without your mind.

This evil entity does not break in with a lot of commotion or noise. It sneaks in silently and progressively steals one memory or thought at a time until it robs a person of his or her identity. The victims of its crimes may actually laugh at the first few attacks, thinking, "How silly of me to forget where I put my keys," or "Why in the world would I have forgotten to turn left at the corner to get to my daughter's house?"

By the time friends and relatives begin to notice such robbery, this mind burglar has entrenched itself so firmly in the affected mind that it is impossible to get it to release its tightening grip. The villain continues the process of gradually stripping that person's thoughts and memories. The best thing loved ones can do is to try to identify the culprit early, arm themselves with information and courage, and try to manage the impending deterioration.

I wrote this book about my experiences with my mother, and subsequently my husband, to help those struggling with the difficult decisions related to caring for someone suffering from dementia. My hope is to give others in this situation the information that I wish I had when I needed it most. Perhaps I can save someone from endless hours of self-recrimination and guilt. Or, just let you know you are not alone. In this book, and on the download kit included with it, you'll find some tools to use when considering care options for loved ones with dementia so you feel like you can make an informed decision.

Please note that I am not a trained medical person. I am just someone who has lived this experience twice, and I want to share it with others. I also want you to know that you can get through this period by looking at things through a different perspective. While I don't suggest wearing rose-colored glasses or being overly optimistic, seeing events with a slight pink tinge will never hurt.

> According to Functional Neuromodulation, Ltd., "Alzheimer's is a progressively debilitating disease that slowly destroys memory and thinking skills, ultimately resulting in death. Alzheimer's is the most common cause of dementia among older persons, affecting 13 percent over age 64 and nearly 50 percent over 85. In 2015 an estimated 5.9 million North Americans suffered from Alzheimer's. The number is expected to exceed 9 million by 2030 and 16 million by 2050. The cost of Alzheimer's to society in North America will exceed $200 billion this year."

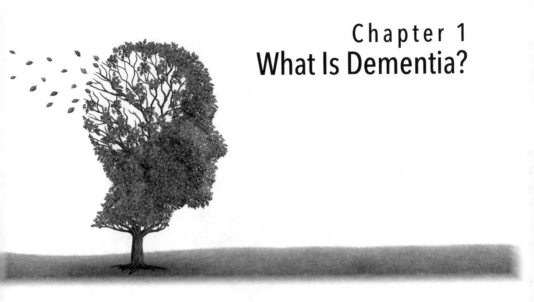

Chapter 1
What Is Dementia?

If you are reading this book you probably have done some of the same research that I have to find out what exactly this disease, dementia, is. You have also most likely asked the same question I did: Does my loved one have dementia or something else with similar symptoms?

The best explanation I have found is that dementia is not a specific disease. The term instead describes a wide range of symptoms associated with a decline in memory or other thinking skills, severe enough to reduce a person's ability to perform everyday activities.

Alzheimer's disease accounts for the greatest percentage of cases of dementia and vascular dementia, which often occurs after a stroke and is the second most common type of dementia (according to the Alzheimer Society of Canada). But many other conditions can cause symptoms similar to dementia, including some that are reversible, such as thyroid problems and vitamin deficiencies. I will discuss these diseases in a bit more detail in Chapters 2 and 3.

According to the Alzheimer's Association, dementia is often incorrectly referred to as "senility" or "senile dementia," which reflects the formerly widespread but incorrect belief that serious mental decline is a normal part of aging. Many people retain their clear thinking and remembering abilities well into old age, and some types of dementia are diagnosed at much younger ages than we would consider "senile" age groups.

If you are concerned that you or a loved one may be experiencing any kind of dementia or mental issue, it is likely time to see a healthcare professional. I have included Checklist 1 here and on the download kit as well. It is a list of questions. If most are answered yes, it should point you in the direction of a qualified healthcare professional for a proper diagnosis. If you decide it is time to see a professional, Checklist 2, available on the download kit as well, can be filled out and brought with you to help you remember what you want to ask.

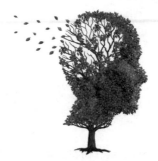

Battle tip: Dementia is not a one-diagnosis-fits-all disease. Don't ignore symptoms or rely solely on a checklist in a book; if you think someone is showing signs of difficulty handling daily living, get him or her to see a doctor for a qualified diagnosis as soon as you can.

Checklist 1
SHOULD YOU OR YOUR LOVED ONE VISIT A DOCTOR ABOUT POSSIBLE DEMENTIA?

☐ Is there significant memory loss?

☐ If yes, is memory worse than previously noted?

☐ Are questions, statements, or stories repeated in the same day?

☐ Are appointments missed or special events forgotten?

☐ Are items misplaced so that they cannot be located?

☐ When items are misplaced are others accused of hiding them or stealing them?

☐ Is there a problem frequently knowing the day, date, month, year, or time? Is there a need to check these things more than once a day?

☐ Is there a problem with getting disoriented in unfamiliar places?

☐ Does confusion increase when outside the home or when traveling?

☐ Is there a problem handling money (tips, calculating change)?

☐ Is there trouble paying bills or doing finances?

☐ Is there a problem with remembering to take medicines or tracking medications taken?

☐ Is there difficulty driving or is the person in question frequently getting lost?

☐ Is using standard appliances (e.g. microwave, oven, stove, remote control, telephone, alarm clock) becoming more difficult?

☐ Are home repair or other home-related tasks such as housekeeping becoming more difficult?

☐ Has participation in usual hobbies such as golf, dancing, exercise, or crafts been reduced?

☐ In familiar surroundings, such as the known neighborhood, are there frequent occasions of getting confused or lost?

☐ Is there a decreased sense of direction?

☐ Is there a problem finding words other than names?

☐ Are the names of family members or friends often confused?

☐ Is there a problem recognizing familiar people?

This questionnaire is not intended to replace a professional diagnosis and you are advised to seek a medical opinion from your healthcare professional in relation to the answers on this questionnaire.

Checklist 2
PREPARING TO VISIT THE DOCTOR

If it's time to visit your healthcare professional, before you go, think through why you're going, what you want to remember to say or ask the doctor, and what you hope to accomplish. Take this checklist with you so you remember to ask all the questions you need.

Describe your reasons for being there:

_____

_____

What health, memory, or mood changes have been observed?

_____

_____

How has/have these thing(s) changed?

_____

_____

When did you first notice the change(s)?

_____

How often does this happen – daily? weekly?

_____

Is there a certain time of day that these changes occur?

_____

What is your response to these things happening? E.g., Anger? Sadness? Frustration?

_____

_____

What activities remain the same? E.g., Ability to pick out clothes and get dressed? Ability to complete a crossword puzzle?

_____

_____

Is there a problem with any of the following? Please check the answers.

Repeating or asking the same thing over and over

☐ Not at all ☐ Sometimes ☐ Frequently ☐ Does not apply

Remembering important events – family birthdays, appointments, holidays

☐ Not at all ☐ Sometimes ☐ Frequently ☐ Does not apply

Handling financial matters – writing cheques, paying bills on time and not duplicating payments

☐ Not at all ☐ Sometimes ☐ Frequently ☐ Does not apply

Taking medications as directed

☐ Not at all ☐ Sometimes ☐ Frequently ☐ Does not apply

Ability to shop for groceries or clothes independently

☐ Not at all ☐ Sometimes ☐ Frequently ☐ Does not apply

Getting lost while driving or walking in a place that is familiar

☐ Not at all ☐ Sometimes ☐ Frequently ☐ Does not apply

Take with you a list of all current medications and other health supplements or vitamins. Also list current medical conditions, e.g., high blood pressure, etc. Provide a list of all past medical conditions, surgeries and hospital stays.

Things to ask the doctor:

What tests will be given and by whom (current doctor or specialist)?

What treatments are available for dementia?

Is there anything else I should know?

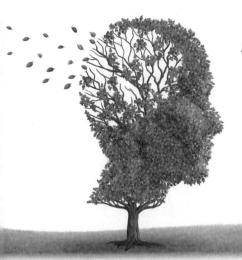

Chapter 2
Alzheimer's Disease

As previously mentioned, Alzheimer's Disease is the most common type of dementia. There is not even a proven test to say that someone has Alzheimer's until after the person is dead and the brain can be examined. But doctors can diagnose symptoms of the disease and say with some certainty that this is what someone is suffering from at an earlier stage.

Early symptoms that indicate dementia related to Alzheimer's include difficulty remembering names and recent events, apathy, and depression. Later symptoms include impaired judgment, disorientation, confusion, behavioral changes, and difficulty speaking, swallowing, and walking.

New criteria and guidelines for diagnosing Alzheimer's were published in 2011 by the National Institute on Aging/Alzheimer's Association. They recommend that Alzheimer's disease be considered a disease with three stages.

- **First stage:** This is sometimes referred to as the "mild" or "early" stage of cognitive impairment. In this stage it may be difficult to pinpoint a problem, as the person with mild Alzheimer's may still be driving and working and still interacting socially with others. The person in this stage would begin to notice memory lapses and the inability to remember recent conversations and events. He or she may not be able to remember some words or names. Tasks the person was once able to do with ease may now be more difficult. The steps to performing a task may not be clear or might be difficult to follow in order. Repeating questions several times in a short period of time, even if previously answered, is another symptom that occurs at this stage. Forgetting what has just been read and losing and misplacing objects are other signs that something is happening. She may have trouble planning and organizing and need reminders for daily activities. He may not be able to react effectively when driving or may have difficulty finding a route he should know well. People at this stage sometimes suffer from depression and experience increased mood swings. This first stage can last anywhere from two to four years.

- **Second stage:** This stage is referred to as the "moderate" or "middle" stage. The person with dementia can no longer hide challenges from others. Memory loss is more severe, and he cannot remember events that just occurred or facts about his personal history. She may not be able to identify family members or friends. He may be unable to recall his own address or telephone number and could get lost going for a walk in his own neighborhood. In socially or mentally challenging situations, she may become moody or withdrawn. Personality and behavioral changes, including becoming suspicious or thinking something has occurred that has not, are symptoms of this stage. A person at this stage will usually require assistance in finding the proper clothing for the occasion or weather. Sleep patterns could change with the person becoming restless at night or sleeping more during the day. For some, mobility and coordination is affected by slowness or other physical symptoms, such as tremors or rigidity.

  At this stage the person is often confused about what day it is or where they are. She may experience bladder or bowel control issues. A person in this stage needs constant reminders, structure in his or her life, and assistance with the activities of daily living. This stage is the longest stage, requires a higher level of care than the first stage, and can last for anywhere from a few to ten years.

- **Third stage:** This last stage is often referred to as "severe" or "late-stage" dementia. During this final stage of the disease, the person will require full-time assistance with daily activities and personal care. He or she has lost the ability to differentiate between current and past experiences and may not recognize surroundings. His verbal and physical skills are deteriorating. She may lose the ability to walk, sit, and eventually swallow. There can be extreme problems with mood and behavior at this stage, and patients are unable to care for themselves. Along with incontinence comes vulnerability to infections and other illnesses. This stage can last up to three years.

You may hear your medical professional talk about a diagnostic framework with more levels within the three stages described. I think this is an attempt to define even further the progression through various stages. While some people decline rapidly and progress quickly through the stages, there is quite a variance in the length of time people diagnosed with dementia can live with the disease. People who are diagnosed in their 70s tend to live longer than people who are diagnosed at age 85 or older. People in the early stage at diagnosis tend to live longer than people in the late stage at diagnosis. Women with Alzheimer's tend to live longer than men who have it. It should be noted that going through these stages usually takes 8 to 10 years, but could stretch out as long as 20 years or more. The overall health and fitness of the person diagnosed can certainly be a factor in longevity.

The Global Deterioration Scale, also known as the Reisberg Scale, includes the following stages:

- **Stage 1:** No impairment. Memory and cognitive abilities appear normal.

- **Stage 2:** Minimal impairment/normal forgetfulness. Memory lapses and changes in thinking are rarely detected by friends, family, or medical personnel, especially as about half of all people over 65 begin noticing problems in concentration and word recall.

- **Stage 3:** Early confusional/mild cognitive impairment. While subtle difficulties begin to impact function, the person may consciously or subconsciously try to cover up his or her problems. Difficulty with retrieving words, planning, organization, misplacing objects, and forgetting recent learning can affect life at home and work. Depression and other changes in mood can also occur. Duration: two to seven years.

- **Stage 4**: Late confusional/mild Alzheimer's. Problems handling finances result from mathematical challenges. Recent events and conversations are increasingly forgotten, although most people in this stage still know themselves and their family. Problems carrying out sequential tasks, including cooking, driving, ordering food at restaurants, and shopping. Often withdraw from social situations, become defensive, and deny problems. Accurate diagnosis of Alzheimer's disease is possible at this stage. Lasts roughly two years.

- **Stage 5**: Early dementia/moderate Alzheimer's disease. Decline is more severe and requires assistance. No longer able to manage independently or recall personal history details and contact information. Frequently disoriented regarding place and or time. People in this stage experience a severe decline in numerical abilities and judgment skills, which can leave them vulnerable to scams and at risk from safety issues. Basic daily living tasks like eating and dressing require increased supervision. Duration: an average of one and a half years.

- **Stage 6**: Middle dementia/moderately severe Alzheimer's disease. Total lack of awareness of present events and inability to accurately remember the past. People in this stage progressively lose the ability to take care of daily living activities like dressing, toileting, and eating but are still able to respond to nonverbal stimuli, and communicate pleasure and pain via behavior. Agitation and hallucinations often show up in the late afternoon or evening. Dramatic personality changes such as wandering or suspicion of family members are common. Many can't remember close family members, but know they are familiar. Lasts approximately two and a half years.

- **Stage 7**: Late or severe dementia and failure to thrive. In this final stage, speech becomes severely limited, as well as the ability to walk or sit. Total support around the clock is needed for all functions of daily living and care. Duration is impacted by quality of care and average length is one to two and a half years.

No matter which system of evaluation that you use or are told about, the disease of Alzheimer's is a steady progression of decline that ultimately leads to the death of someone with the disease. At this point there is no cure although there are medications that have been suggested to ease the symptoms of memory loss and confusion for a limited amount of time.

All of the current drugs approved in North America for the treatment of mild to moderate dementia are from a class of drugs called cholinesterase inhibitors. They prevent the breakdown of acetylcholine (chemical messenger in the brain) which is a substance that is necessary to support communication between nerve cells. Keeping these levels high for a period of time can improve memory, language, judgement, and other thought processes, but they are only effective from 6 to 12 months on average for only about one half of the people that they are prescribed for.

Menatine is another drug that is FDA approved for treatment of moderate to severe dementia. It regulates the activity of glutamate, another chemical in the brain that affects learning and memory. Once again, this is not a cure and does not work for everyone and is also not effective over a long period.

Table 1
COMMON DRUGS USED FOR DEMENTIA

Generic	Brand	Approved For	Side Effects
donepezil	Aricept	All stages	Nausea, vomiting, loss of appetite, and increased frequency of bowel movements
galantamine	Razadyne	Mild to moderate	Nausea, vomiting, loss of appetite, and increased frequency of bowel movements
memantine	Namenda	Moderate to severe	Headache, constipation, confusion, and dizziness
rivastigmine	Exelon	Mild to moderate	Nausea, vomiting, loss of appetite, and increased frequency of bowel movements
memantine + donepezil	Namzaric	Moderate to severe	Headache, diarrhea, dizziness, loss of appetite, vomiting, nausea, and bruising

There are several alternative treatments that are being promoted and advertised as potential treatments for dementia but they are mostly based on personal testimonies or some sort of tradition-based information. Some have a small amount of scientific research that has been conducted but they have not necessarily undergone extensive scientific testing and evaluation. Things like coconut oil, coenzyme Q10, coral calcium, gingko biloba, huperzine A (Chinese moss extract), omega 3, and tramiprosate (natural seaweed extract) may be promoted as medical foods that will enhance memory or delay the onset of dementia but, to date, have not undergone the rigorous studies a prescription drug must go through.

There are currently many studies being done to promote and develop new drugs for the treatment of dementia. Most of them are targeting the brain changes that are the underlying cause of dementia and not just treating the symptoms. It is hoped that there will be some effective drug or combination of drugs that can assist in preventing dementia in the future.

Things that have been shown to decrease cardiovascular disease may be helpful in decreasing the potential for developing dementia. Things like regular exercise and a heart-healthy diet could, for example, help protect against the onset of dementia. Maintaining social networks and keeping mentally active are also talked about as potential delaying factors. Serious head trauma has also been linked to the development of dementia so protecting your head in vulnerable situations is advised.

1. Signs and Symptoms of Alzheimer's Disease

For many people, detecting the first signs of memory problems in themselves or a family member brings an immediate fear of Alzheimer's disease. However, most people over 65 experience some level of forgetfulness. It is normal for age-related brain shrinkage to produce changes in processing speed, attention, and short-term memory, creating so-called "senior moments." Forgetfulness is merely inconvenient, though, and generally involves unimportant information. Understanding the significance of these age-related changes begins with knowing the difference between what is normal and what is an early symptom of Alzheimer's.

2. Alzheimer's versus Normal Aging

How can you tell if someone has Alzheimer's disease, or whether his or her memory problems are just a natural part of aging? The examples in the following sections show the difference between normal aging and what could be considered a more serious form of deterioration.

2.1 Memory loss that disrupts daily life

One of the most common signs of Alzheimer's is memory loss, especially forgetting recently learned information. Others include forgetting important dates or events, asking for the same information over and over, and increasingly needing to rely on memory aids (e.g., reminder notes or electronic devices) or family members for things that the person used to handle on his or her own.

2.1a What's a typical age-related change?

It is typical for an aging person to sometimes forget names or appointments, but remember them later or when someone tells him or her about it.

2.2 Challenges in planning or solving problems

Some people with Alzheimer's may experience changes in the ability to develop and follow a plan or work with numbers. He may have trouble following a familiar recipe or keeping track of monthly bills. She may have difficulty concentrating and take much longer to do things than before.

2.2a What's a typical age-related change?

It is typical for an aging person to make occasional errors when balancing a checkbook, or have to slow down a task or follow notes for something that used to be done with ease.

2.3 Difficulty completing familiar tasks at home, at work, or at leisure

People with Alzheimer's often find it hard to complete daily tasks. They may have trouble driving to a familiar location, managing a budget at work, or remembering the rules of a favorite game. Using a computer may become difficult even though it used to be easy.

2.3a What's a typical age-related change?

It is typical for an aging person to occasionally need help to use the settings on a microwave or to record a television show.

2.4 Confusion with time or place

People with Alzheimer's can lose track of dates, seasons, and the passage of time. They may have trouble understanding something if it is not happening immediately. Sometimes they forget where they are or how they got there.

2.4a What's a typical age-related change?

It is typical for an aging person to become confused about the day of the week but figure it out later, or make a wrong turn but realize that it was a mistake.

2.5 Trouble understanding visual images and spatial relationships

For some people, vision problems are a sign of Alzheimer's. They may have difficulty reading, judging distance, and determining color or contrast, which may cause problems with driving. Stopping far too soon for a stop sign or stopping past the stop line consistently are other examples of how you might see this symptom manifest.

2.5a What's a typical age-related change?

It is typical for an aging person to experience vision changes related to cataracts or needing a new prescription. These can be corrected through surgery or with glasses.

2.6 New problems with words in speaking or writing

People with Alzheimer's may have trouble following or joining a conversation. They may stop in the middle of a conversation and have no idea how to continue or they may repeat themselves. They may struggle with vocabulary, have problems finding the right word, or call things by the wrong name (e.g., call a "watch" a "hand-clock"). The other day, my husband asked if he looked "presidential" when he actually meant "presentable." (On the other hand, maybe he wanted to look like a president!)

2.6a What's a typical age-related change?

It is typical for an aging person to sometimes have trouble finding the right word, but ultimately find it.

2.7 Misplacing things and losing the ability to retrace steps

A person with Alzheimer's disease may put things in unusual places. He or she may lose things and be unable to retrace his or her steps to find them. He may accuse others of stealing, and this may occur more frequently over time. My husband often puts the groceries away in very strange places, like the milk in the cupboard and the cereal in the fridge.

2.7a What's a typical age-related change?

It is typical for an aging person to misplace things from time to time and need to retrace steps to find them.

2.8 Decreased or poor judgment

People with Alzheimer's may experience changes in judgment or decision-making. For example, they may use poor judgment when dealing with money, giving large amounts to telemarketers. They may pay less attention to grooming or keeping themselves clean. I have to remind my husband to take a shower or to shave, and he is always taking out his wallet when we go somewhere, thinking that he must pay for something even when I tell him that it's already been paid for. If I were not with him, someone could take advantage of him by having him pay for something more than once.

2.8a What's a typical age-related change?

It is typical for an aging person to make a bad decision once in a while, but recognize that it was a bad decision.

2.9 Withdrawal from work or social activities

A person with Alzheimer's may start to remove himself or herself from hobbies, social activities, work projects, or sports. He may have trouble keeping up with a favorite sports team or remembering how to complete a favorite hobby. She may also avoid being social because of the changes they have experienced. For example, following a conversation is more difficult, and he may be more sensitive to noise.

2.9a What's a typical age-related change?

It is typical for an aging person to occasionally feel weary of work, family, and social obligations.

2.10 Changes in mood and personality

The moods and personalities of people with Alzheimer's can change over time. He can become confused, suspicious, depressed, fearful, or anxious. She may be easily upset at home, at work, with friends, or in places where she is out of her comfort zone.

2.10a What's a typical age-related change?

It is typical for an aging person to develop very specific ways of doing things and become irritable when a routine is disrupted.

Note: If you think that someone is showing signs of Alzheimer's disease, please ensure that you take him or her to a qualified person to be tested.

If you are the kind of person who prefers simple lists, the Alzheimer Society of Canada has developed the graphic in Figure 1, that we have reprinted with their permission.

1. Memory loss affecting day-to-day abilities: forgetting things often or struggling to retain new information.

2. Difficulty performing familiar tasks: forgetting how to do something you've been doing your whole life, such as preparing a meal or getting dressed.

3. Problems with language: forgetting words or substituting words that don't fit the context.

4. Disorientation in time and space: not knowing what day of the week it is or getting lost in a familiar place.

5. Impaired judgment: not recognizing a medical problem that needs attention or wearing light clothing on a cold day.

6. Problems with abstract thinking: not understanding what numbers signify on a calculator, for example, or how they're used.

7. Misplacing things: putting things in strange places, like an iron in the freezer or a wristwatch in the sugar bowl.

8. Changes in mood and behavior: exhibiting severe mood swings from being easygoing to quick-tempered.

9. Changes in personality: behaving out of character such as feeling paranoid or threatened.

10. Loss of initiative: losing interest in friends, family, and favorite activities.

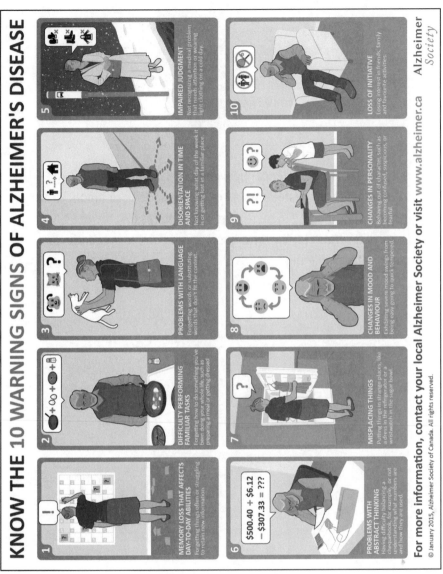

Figure 1: Know the 10 Warning Signs of Alzheimer's Disease

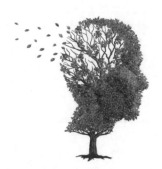

Battle tip: The differences between normal aging and Alzheimer's can be determined by comparing the common symptoms of aging to more serious symptoms that disrupt daily life. Watch for the ten signs that can point to dementia versus normal aging.

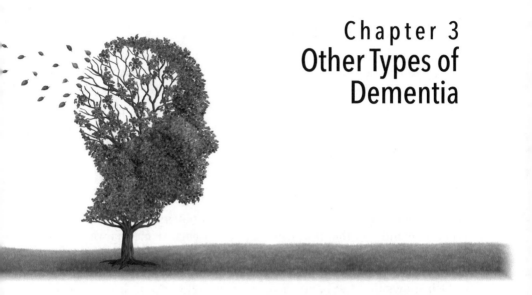

Chapter 3
Other Types of Dementia

We know that dementia symptoms can be symptoms of disorders other than Alzheimer's disease. This chapter briefly describes the most common types of dementia, the symptoms related to them, and how scientists have recorded the brain changes related to each type in order to recognize them.

It is important to read about the various types of dementia so you are aware of the many forms this illness can take. Not all dementias are age-related dementia and there are a number of treatable conditions that produce symptoms similar to dementia. These can include some vitamin and hormone deficiencies, stress, depression, pain, chronic illness, alcohol abuse, infections, and brain tumors. That is why it is so important to contact a physician when there are major changes in memory. Those changes should be taken seriously, not just considered normal.

The following sections outline types of dementia that aren't Alzheimer's, in a very basic fashion. For more information about these types of dementia please consult your physician and other reputable sources.

1. Vascular Dementia

Previously known as multi-infarct or post-stroke dementia, vascular dementia is less common as a sole cause of dementia than Alzheimer's, accounting for about 10 percent of dementia cases.

1.1 Symptoms of vascular dementia

Impaired judgment or ability to make decisions, plan, or organize is more likely to be the initial symptom, as opposed to the memory loss often associated with the initial symptoms of Alzheimer's. This occurs from blood vessel blockage or damage leading to infarcts (strokes) or bleeding in the brain. The location, number, and size of the brain injury determines how the individual's thinking and physical functioning are affected.

1.2 Brain changes in people with vascular dementia

Brain imaging can often detect blood vessel problems implicated in vascular dementia. In the past, evidence for vascular dementia was used to exclude a diagnosis of Alzheimer's disease (and vice versa). That practice is no longer considered consistent with pathologic evidence, which shows that the brain changes of several types of dementia can be present simultaneously. When any two or more types of dementia are present at the same time, the individual is considered to have "mixed dementia" (see section 4).

2. Dementia with Lewy Bodies (DLB)

2.1 Symptoms of DLB

People with dementia with lewy bodies (DLB; also referred to as Lewy Body Dementia or LBD) often have memory loss and thinking problems common in Alzheimer's, but are more likely than people with Alzheimer's to have initial or early symptoms such as sleep disturbances; well-formed visual hallucinations; and slowness, gait imbalance, or other parkinsonian movement features. This disease is named after Frederick H. Lewy, MD, the neurologist who discovered the alpha-synuclein protein, the chief component of Lewy bodies, while working in Dr. Alois Alzheimer's laboratory during the early 1900s.

2.2 Brain changes in those with DLB

Lewy bodies are abnormal aggregations (or clumps) of the protein alpha-synuclein. When they develop in a part of the brain called the cortex, dementia can result. Alpha-synuclein also aggregates in the brains of people with Parkinson's disease, but the aggregates may appear in a pattern that is different from DLB.

The brain changes of dementia with Lewy bodies alone can cause dementia, or they can be present at the same time as the brain changes of Alzheimer's disease and/or vascular dementia, with each abnormality contributing to the development of dementia. When this happens, the individual is said to have mixed dementia (see section 4.).

3. Parkinson's Disease

In some cases, as Parkinson's disease progresses, it results in a progressive dementia similar to dementia with Lewy bodies or Alzheimer's. The same "Lewy bodies" or alpha-synuclein protein clumps are found in the person with Parkinson's disease. The primary difference is that Parkinson's disease is found initially in the part of the brain that controls movement and then slowly spreads to the other parts of the brain. There have been found in Parkinson's patients the plaques and tangles associated with Alzheimer's as well as the Lewy bodies. If a person is diagnosed with movement issues and then a year, or more, later with dementia issues he or she is considered to have Parkinson's dementia. If people display the movement issues at the same time as the dementia then the dementia is diagnosed as Lewy body dementia, or if they are diagnosed with Lewy body dementia and then movement issues within a year of the dementia diagnoses, they are considered Lewy body dementia patients.

3.1 Symptoms of Parkinson's disease

Problems with movement are a common symptom early in the disease. If dementia develops, symptoms are often similar to dementia with Lewy bodies. Not all Parkinson's patients develop dementia.

3.2 Brain changes in those with Parkinson's disease

Alpha-synuclein clumps are likely to begin in an area deep in the brain called the *substantia nigra*. These clumps are thought to cause degeneration of the nerve cells that produce dopamine. Dopamine functions as a neurotransmitter that sends signals to other nerve cells involved in motor control.

4. Mixed Dementia

In mixed dementia, abnormalities linked to more than one cause of dementia occur simultaneously in the brain. Recent studies suggest that mixed dementia is more common than previously thought. Most people with mixed dementia are diagnosed and treated for the type of dementia that they are first thought to have, i.e., if diagnosed with Alzheimer's then they are treated as if that is the only dementia they have. It has been said that more than half of the people diagnosed with Alzheimer's many have some form of mixed dementia but it cannot be diagnosed except by an autopsy on the brain.

4.1 Symptoms of mixed dementia

Mixed dementia symptoms may vary, depending on the types of brain changes involved and the brain regions affected. In many cases, symptoms may be similar to or even indistinguishable from those of Alzheimer's or another type of dementia. In other cases, a person's symptoms may suggest that more than one type of dementia is present.

4.2 Brain changes in those with mixed dementia

Mixed dementia is characterized by the hallmark abnormalities of more than one cause of dementia, most commonly, Alzheimer's and vascular dementia, but also other types, such as dementia with Lewy bodies.

5. Frontotemporal Dementia

Frontotemporal dementia includes dementias such as:

- **Behavioral variant FTD (bvFTD):** This condition is where the nerve cell loss is most prominent in the areas that control conduct, judgment, empathy, and foresight.

- **Primary progressive aphasia (PPA):** The second major form of this type of dementia affects language skills, speaking, writing, and comprehension. There are two forms of this PPA where individuals lose the ability to understand or formulate words in a spoken sentence, or, where a person's speech is very hesitant, labored, or grammatically incorrect.

- **Pick's disease:** In 1892 Dr. Arnold Pick identified a patient with distinct symptoms affecting language. Some doctors still use this term to describe FTD.

- **Corticobasal degeneration:** This is where arms and legs become uncoordinated or stiff.

- **Progressive supranuclear palsy:** This is what describes muscle stiffness, difficulty walking, and changes in posture, and also affects eye movement.

- **Amyotrophic Lateral Sclerosis (ALS):** This causes muscle weakness or wasting. It is a motor neuron disease also known as Lou Gehrig's disease.

5.1 Symptoms of frontotemporal dementia (FTD)

Typical symptoms of frontotemporal dementia include changes in personality and behavior and difficulty with language. Nerve cells in the front and side regions of the brain are especially affected. In about one third of all cases of FTD degenerations are inherited. Genetic counseling and testing is available now on individuals with family histories of FTD. There are no known risk factors known other than a family history.

5.2 Brain changes in those with frontotemporal dementia

No distinguishing microscopic abnormality is linked to all cases in people with frontotemporal dementia. People with FTD generally develop symptoms at a younger age (at about age 60) and survive for fewer years than those with Alzheimer's.

6. Creutzfeldt-Jakob Disease (CJD)

Creutzfeldt-Jakob disease (CJD) is the most common human form of a group of rare, fatal brain disorders affecting people and certain other mammals. The main types of CJD are identified as:

- Sporadic CJD, spontaneously developed for no known reason and accounts for 85 percent of the cases.

- Familial CJD, a hereditary form of the disease which accounts for 10 to 15 percent of the cases.

- Acquired CJD, resulting from exposure to an external source of the abnormal prion protein. These cases account for about 1 percent of the cases and could be caused by medical procedures involving instruments used in neurosurgery.

- Variant CJD ("mad cow disease") occurs in cattle, and has been transmitted to people who consumed beef from cattle whose feed included processed brain tissue from other animals.

6.1 Symptoms of CJD

CJD is a rapidly fatal disorder that impairs memory and coordination, and causes behavioral changes. Depression and agitation, apathy and mood swings along with rapidly worsening confusion, disorientation, and problems with memory, thinking, and judgment occur. Also difficulty walking and muscle stiffness, twitches, and involuntary jerky movements occur.

6.2 Brain changes in those with CJD

CJD results from misfolded prion protein that causes a domino effect, in which prion protein throughout the brain misfolds and thus malfunctions. The prion protein is found throughout the body but its normal function is not yet known and it begins to shape itself into a three-dimensional shape which triggers the prion proteins in the brain to also fold into this abnormal shape. Scientists do not know why this three-dimensional shape of the prion protein starts to destroy brain cells.

7. Normal Pressure Hydrocephalus (NPH)

This is a brain disorder in which excess cerebrospinal fluid accumulates in the brain's ventricles, which are hollow, fluid-filled chambers. NPH is called "normal pressure" because despite the excess fluid found in the ventricles, the cerebrospinal fluid pressure measured during a spinal tap is often normal. As the ventricles fill up with fluid, they can disrupt and damage nearby brain tissue.

In some cases, normal pressure hydrocephalus is caused by other brain disorders such as hemorrhages, infections, or inflammation. But in most cases, the fluid buildup happens for unknown reasons.

7.1 Symptoms of normal pressure hydrocephalus

Symptoms of NPH include difficulty walking, memory loss, and inability to control urination.

7.2 Brain changes in those with normal pressure hydrocephalus

This disease is caused by the buildup of fluid in the brain, so it can sometimes be corrected with surgical installation of a shunt in the brain to drain excess fluid. Shunting does not work for everyone and there is currently no known effective cure for NPH.

8. Huntington's disease

Huntington's disease is an inherited, progressive brain disorder caused by a single defective gene on chromosome 4. Most people with Huntington's disease develop signs and symptoms in their 30s or 40s, but the onset of disease may be earlier or later in life. When disease onset begins before age 20, the condition is called juvenile Huntington's disease. Earlier onset often results in a somewhat different presentation of symptoms and faster disease progression.

8.1 Symptoms of Huntington's disease

Symptoms of Huntington's include abnormal involuntary movements, a severe decline in thinking and reasoning skills, irritability, depression, and other mood changes.

8.2 Brain changes in those with Huntington's disease

The gene defect in Huntington's causes abnormalities in a brain protein that, over time, lead to worsening symptoms.

9. Wernicke-Korsakoff syndrome

Wernicke-Korsakoff syndrome is a chronic memory disorder caused by severe deficiency of thiamine (vitamin B1). The most common cause is alcohol abuse.

9.1 Symptoms of Wernicke-Korsakoff syndrome

Memory problems in those with Wernicke-Korsakoff syndrome may be strikingly severe while other thinking and social skills seem relatively unaffected.

9.2 Brain changes in those with Wernicke-Korskoff syndrome

Thiamine helps brain cells produce energy from sugar. When thiamine levels fall too low, brain cells cannot generate enough energy to function properly.

10. Dementia Is Not a One-Diagnosis-Fits-All Disease

If you made it through this chapter, congratulations! I realize that there is a lot of information here and elsewhere about the various types of dementia, but I want you to be aware of the vastness of these diseases and how any single type of dementia or a combination of more than one type can literally infiltrate people's minds in numerous ways.

I hope that you recognize that there are many underlying causes of dementia. It is not a one-diagnosis-fits-all type of disease.

The most important thing I can say is this: If you think someone you know is showing symptoms of any of the diseases mentioned, please take him or her to a doctor for a qualified diagnosis.

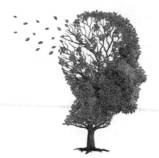

Battle tip: Although Alzheimer's is the most common form of dementia, estimated to relate to 60 to 80 percent of cases, there are many other types. There is also a category called mixed dementia in which a person displays symptoms of several different diseases. Knowing the symptoms of each type can help you help your loved one.

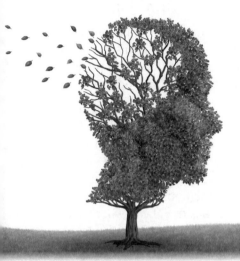

Chapter 4
My Story:
My Mother and
Signs of Dementia

My first battle with dementia began with my mother. I imagine that the majority of people think of their mothers as brilliant and beautiful and among the smartest people in the world. That was definitely how I felt about mine.

I hope that some of her talents were passed down to me, but I am very sure that many of them were passed along to her granddaughters and great-granddaughters.

Perhaps my story will resonate with others who feel the same way about their mothers or other loved ones — about how such a talented person became a victim of the vicious villain named dementia. My story is just one of many sorrowful tales of people who are struggling with a loved one developing dementia. These stories do not have happy endings, but I hope that you will discover that we can learn to love and accept our loved ones through the changes in their lives, even when these changes are not what we wished for them, or for ourselves.

Let me tell you about my mother.

My mother was an avid knitter until dementia took that skill away from her. She could knit while she read a book or watched a TV program, and it always amazed me how the balls of wool would seem to automatically transform themselves into warm sweaters, mittens, hats, and blankets. One of my favorite childhood memories is picking out which Siwash sweater she would knit for me that year. Would it be the one with the kittens on it? Or should I go for a pattern with horses?

My mother was also a very creative crochet expert, and new items were always popping up to decorate the house. Along this same line, she did many needlework and petit-point projects. Some of my most cherished possessions are the works of art that she crafted.

If there was something new that came up in the way of a craft, my mother would try it and usually she did not need detailed instructions; she just figured it out. We had wrapped candy made into Christmas wreaths and coat hangers with brightly colored crochet covers on them to keep clothing items from sliding off the metal. We had macrame hanging planters for almost every plant in the house, and hundreds of sparkling crochet stars shone on our Christmas tree. Everywhere in the house you found evidence of my mother's crafting accomplishments, and every scrap of wool or empty paper tube was transformed into something.

At Christmas, my mother would practice playing the few Christmas songs she knew on the piano, the most notable being "Christmas is Coming and the Geese are Getting Fat," which would waft throughout the house for the month or so before December 25. At first she played hesitantly, with a few false starts and prolonged pauses, but by the time we were asked to sing along around the piano, she had mastered the tunes. Our family was not blessed with wonderful singing voices, so the occasional missed note in my mother's playing probably matched whatever note or key we were singing.

My mother's talents were not limited to enhanced motor skills like typing, shorthand, piano playing, and handicrafts; she used her advanced mental abilities as a very skillful bridge player and learned the intricacies of playing mahjong with her friends. She loved to read a good book and was excellent at crossword puzzles. There was usually music playing on the record player, everything from classical to show tunes. I remember her dancing through the house singing "I'm gonna wash that man right out of my hair" from the musical *South Pacific*. She had an incredible zest for life.

As you can tell, my mother had a very fertile and full mind. It must have been difficult for the dementia, the memory thief, to choose where to start raiding her memories.

Mom's passion for life remained strong even when she was diagnosed with colon cancer and had to wear a colostomy bag for the last 25 years of her life. She never once complained about this situation. She expressed her gratitude that she was able to see her grandchildren grow and even found time to visit others who were about to undergo colostomy operations to give them support and encouragement.

You would have thought that her battle with cancer would have been a big enough challenge for her to face and that she would be spared the battle with an even more onerous foe called dementia. But dementia does not play favorites.

I will be forever grateful for the chance I got to bond again with my mother for a couple of years before dementia stepped in and she forgot who I was. Even though I noticed some peculiar things happening, I cherished the time that I spent with her.

She came to live with me after my father died. At first she seemed fine with continuing her monthly bridge club and volunteering to take the "old folks" from the long-term care facility shopping. These shopping trips were something that she still did even though she was 80 years old herself; older than most of her charges on the shopping excursions.

I began to notice my mother doing things that she had not done before, like leaving an empty coffee pot on the coffee maker with the burner on. This translated into me replacing several glass pots after they cracked from the heat. She also seemed not to notice if a coffee cup was clean or not, and I would often find mugs with coffee still in them sitting in the cupboard.

Her passion for crossword puzzles was diminishing because she just could not think of the correct word for eight across. She would mutter to herself about getting forgetful and, although she was still driving her car, it became a game of "where did I put my car keys?" every time she went out. Sometimes that would escalate to "where did I park my car?" and she would joke about the extra exercise she got looking for her vehicle in the parking lot at a local strip mall.

People would call the house when we were out and she would tell us that someone had called, but she could not remember who it was. She started to write down people's names when they called but soon I could no longer read her writing. Sometimes neither could she.

Although she had a closet full of nice clothes, she began to wear the same outfit several times a week even if it had a few stains on it. Undoubtedly they were coffee stains because I could tell at the end of the day where Mom had travelled through the house—there was a trail of coffee drops wherever she had been.

She started calling me at work to see if I would be home for dinner, and then she'd call again in a few minutes to ask the same question. After I had confirmed I would be home that night for dinner, I would come home and find her frying up an egg for a sandwich. I would ask why she was doing that when I had told her I was about to make dinner. She would say, "Oh, I thought you weren't coming home tonight."

Mom began to pull into the driveway of our house using the "feeler method." We would hear the car scraping along the stucco at the side of the house and my daughter and I would look at each other and say, "I guess Granny is home!"

I was somewhat in denial about her diminishing mental state even after these types of incidents. After all, this was my best friend, my advisor, and the person I thought had all the answers. I easily let myself believe that she was just getting a little forgetful. Don't make that mistake. If you see these symptoms in someone you love, don't gloss over them. Get help.

Eventually I could no longer ignore the signs that she was truly failing mentally and needed more care than I could provide. It was dangerous for her to be driving, for her own safety and the safety of others. I was constantly worried that she would turn on the stove and not remember to turn it off.

In consultation with her doctor and the rest of the family, we soon decided it was necessary to place Mom where she would have care available to her on a continuous basis. I was still working full time and raising my own teenagers, and neither of my siblings was in a position to provide a secure place for Mom. Since she could no longer drive her car, she also needed to be in a more central location that had access to transportation so she could get to her appointments and outings.

The big question — and it was big! — was what type of facility and where?

Eventually, we found what we thought was the perfect place for my mother. An assisted living retirement community, it was a very new building with independent living apartments that each had a bedroom, living room, kitchenette, and senior-friendly bathroom facilities. Mom

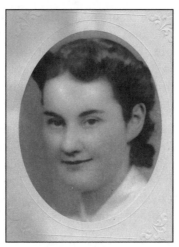

Figure 2: Picture of Mother

could go down each night for a communal supper, and she could prepare her own breakfast and lunch in her apartment if she wished. She also had the option of taking all of her meals in the communal dining room.

The place looked like a very expensive hotel. The hallways had lovely carpet in rich burgundy and gold, and the walls were painted in the same vibrant colors, with a chair railing along each wall. Decorative moldings framed each door and window. The dining room was very elegant, with large windows on two sides, and the tables were set with white tablecloths and linen napkins for every meal. It all gave an impression of dignity and respect.

The retirement community had on-call nursing staff and arranged for people to come in to assist residents with laundry and housekeeping. There were scheduled activities and entertainment that residents could choose to participate in. The front desk was manned 24 hours a day to monitor who came in and out of the building, but the residents' ability to come and go was not restricted.

We moved Mom in. We were able to fit in all of her familiar furniture: her bedroom suite, her favorite chair, a coffee table and desk that belonged to her mother, her wall unit for her television set, many of the paintings she had on the wall in her previous home, and lots of other familiar items. The bedspread and drapes that she loved were also transferred to her suite.

There were many benefits to Mom's new home. As her suite was on the top floor of the building, it was very quiet. There was a lovely balcony, where I put some plants in the summer for her to enjoy. Lots of light poured into the unit to make it seem quite cheery, and the bathroom had a walk-in shower with a seat that she could use when bathing. My mother paid a monthly rental fee that was a bit expensive but manageable. After all, you can't put a price on peace of mind, and security for someone you love.

The first day that we took her to her new residence, I felt like the mother taking her child to camp for the first time. I was thinking, "Will she like it here? Will she make some new friends? Will she be homesick? Will she be happy?" I was bursting with pride when I saw her walk into the dining room by herself, sit at the table she was shown, and begin talking with the other ladies. As I peeked through the curtains to the dining room, I felt that I could leave her and she would be OK.

Initially, Mom seemed to fit into her new environment quite well. When we went to visit we would find her wheeling another resident down to the dining room for lunch or chatting in the games room with the other residents. There was even a bridge game that she took part in going on most afternoons.

She was OK there for a couple of years and it worked out well that she had a number of outside people who would come to assist her. A nurse came to make sure she took her medications and to check on her colostomy and assist her with changing the colostomy bag. A housekeeper came into her apartment and did the cleaning and dusting and took her laundry out to be washed and dried. The residents also checked on each other and made sure that people came down for their meals. Mom went to the activities provided in the facility and some of her old friends would come to visit her. It seemed like this environment was secure and met all her needs. I felt very relieved she was being taken care of and that, as the facility was very close to my workplace, I could stop in at lunch or after work to have a brief visit with her. I always made a point of coming to special events that were held at her residence — the special teas and fashion shows were fun to attend with her. I got to meet and know many of the other residents and they seemed to be a very caring group. I did notice that they sometimes tended to gather in groups and gossip about others outside of the group, but you often see that kind of thing and I didn't worry about it given the other things to consider.

Sadly, at some point those seemingly caring seniors that I just described above developed what I (an obviously emotionally attached daughter) can only describe as a pack mentality. Once they saw weakness in one of their own, they circled around and started nipping at my mom as she declined. I began to get reports that the other residents did not want my mother sitting at their table for meals anymore because they felt that she was not as clean as she should be. They reported that she was going outside without a proper coat for the weather conditions and that she was seen wandering the hallways and entering other people's apartments. She was shunned from the bridge table for failing to play effectively.

The assisted living complex then put a wristband on my mother that would set off an alarm at the front desk anytime she was close to the front door. This embarrassed her greatly and tears would spring into her eyes every time the alarm went off.

"I don't know why I am wearing this thing," she would say.

I was desperate to try and find a way to make her feel OK about having to wear the wristband. I told her that this situation was to keep her safe, or that it was for her own good, but the words sounded hollow even to me as I said them. Sometimes I would try to joke with her and say that the alarm system was to keep the staff manning the front desk on their toes so they would not have to fill out lots of paperwork about losing a resident. Or sometimes I would tell her that the buzzer was to wake up the attendant at the front door. I could not help but think that the bracelet caused, rather than prevented some of the potential problems it was intended to solve, but I do not know that for sure. More important is that my feeling that Mom was in the right place began to diminish, and I had no idea what the next step was, if there was one.

Mom started to refuse to go down to meals and began squirreling away cupcakes and cookies that were left in the coffee area on her floor. She would stash these treasures around her apartment, often just wrapped in a napkin and not necessarily in the fridge where they should have been. We had to have the main circuit breaker for the stove in her unit shut off so she would not leave a burner on. My mother would start to take off her colostomy bag on her own and wonder what that thing was doing attached to her stomach. The nursing staff was there twice daily to explain why she needed it and to help her, and she would seem to understand for a short while.

She lost the ability to make phone calls or even answer the phone if it rang. The people who came to help her with her laundry stated that she was hiding her clothing in mysterious places, such as under the bed. Her ability to write out a check was lost, and even her signature was almost illegible. Her memory had also deteriorated, and she could not tell you what she had for lunch or even if she'd had lunch. The assisted living residence was not equipped for the extended care that my mother now needed, and she started to become somewhat fearful in that environment. The summer camp feeling was over. It was time to move Mom into another type of facility.

I felt concerned and somewhat guilty about putting her into the assisted living complex, but that was nothing compared to the despair I felt when we took her to the long-term care facility. I felt like I was putting her in jail even though she had never committed a crime in her life. All her days had been given to helping others and being a kind, wonderful person, and we were now leaving her in this bland old building where she once again would not know anyone and would be in an unknown environment. I had constant thoughts about quitting my job and spending what would be the rest of my mother's life looking after her. This beautiful woman deserved to be treated in the best possible manner, but I still had commitments to my own children and knew that I did not have the skill or the patience it would take to look after changing her colostomy bag and making sure she was safe 24 hours a day. There was no bursting with pride on leaving her at the long-term care facility—only tears, although it was a necessary move.

Once you're ready to learn about the different types of facilities available for seniors, read Chapter 5.

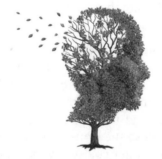

Battle tip: Moving my mother into an assisted living home seemed like the best alternative initially, but as time went on, she needed more intensive care. If you suspect the senior you are looking for a residence for has dementia, it may be a good idea to find a place that offers both assisted living and dementia care so the person does not have to change facilities after a couple of years.

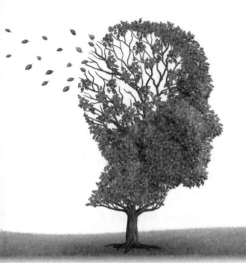

Chapter 5
Living Options for Seniors and Those with Dementia

As people get older, they or their family members may start to consider other, more suitable living arrangements. If someone you care about has some form of dementia, it may be time to consider moving him or her out of the home to a facility where safety and security can be assured unless you have unlimited funds to provide a 24-hour caregiver in the home. People with dementia often have trouble with bathing and normal hygiene activities and so modifications often need to be made to their homes if the consideration is for them to stay there.

Most seniors aged 65 to 70 still live in their own homes and conduct their own affairs. But as the baby boomer population ages, a higher percentage of seniors will move from their homes into some other form of accommodation. See *Aging Safely in Your Home*, another Self-Counsel Press title, for more about this.

There are so many names for different types of residences to choose from that even this first major step can quickly become overwhelming. I found that I was inundated with new terminology and had no idea what it meant. To help you, I will try to lend you some of my understanding of the various terms in this chapter.

With different terminology used across North America, the names for residential care facilities can include lodges, assisted living, supportive housing, long-term care homes, nursing homes, and personal care homes. These facilities offer different levels of care and may be freestanding or co-located with other types of housing, care facilities, or hospitals.

In your search for accommodation, you may come across terms like supportive living, independent living, home care, enhanced supportive living, memory care, extended care, designated assisted living, nursing home, and long-term care. Not only are there a variety of terms, but there are various levels in some types of living arrangements, like DAL4 or Designated Assisted Living Level 4, for example, which is a designation for dementia care residents who tend to wander. There are terms like "secure ward" or "lock-down facility." The latter sounds like a prison to me, but they are residences that control who enters and exits the facility through controls on the door system, either by using buzzers, codes, or locks.

There are various terms for the workers in these facilities too, such as PCAs (personal care attendants), HSWs (home support workers), HCAs (health care aides), LPNs (licensed practical nurses), RNs (registered nurses), ACNPs (acute care nurse practitioners), and RPNs (registered psychiatric nurses). If those aren't enough, there are many other terms as well, but these are the common ones that I encountered in my search for a place for my mother.

After sorting through all the verbiage, I discovered that the types of accommodation for aging seniors fall into three main categories: independent living, assisted/supportive living, and long-term care/facility living.

1. Independent Living

As you can guess from the title, people living independently continue to live in their own space, prepare their own meals, and take care of their own hygiene. This remains an option for them because they typically do not have special or acute mobility needs. This type of living can continue on in the senior's own home, and it allows what is sometimes described as "aging in place." Another type of independent living for seniors is facilities designed for this purpose.

1.1 Aging in place

Staying at home offers the advantage of keeping the senior person in a familiar place where he or she knows the neighbors and the community. A wide range of home care services are available to help seniors maintain their independence within the comfort of their own homes, from in-home care to day programs. Transportation systems like DATS (Disabled Adults Transfer Service) in Canada or privately run senior transportation services, such as Driving Miss Daisy, can make traveling out of the house easier. Home repairs or modifications to make a senior's life easier and safer, such as installing a wheelchair ramp, bathtub railings, or emergency response system are available and, in some cases, funding can be obtained from government sources to make these modifications affordable.

Staying at home may be a good option if:

- The senior has a close network of nearby family, friends, and neighbors.
- Transportation is easily accessible, including alternate transportation to driving.
- The neighborhood is safe.
- The home can be modified to reflect changing needs.
- Any home and yard maintenance is not overwhelming or can be outsourced.
- Physical and medical needs do not require a high level of care.
- The senior does not suffer from dementia and is willing and able to reach out for social support.

Aging in place is a less effective senior housing option once mobility or mental acuity is limited. Being unable to leave your home frequently and socialize with others can lead to isolation, loneliness, and depression. So, even if aging in place seems like a good idea today, it's important to have a plan for the future when needs may change and staying at home may no longer be the best option.

1.2 Living in a retirement community

Independent living accommodations can range from luxury communities with lots of amenities, such as golf courses and gourmet dining facilities, to simpler complexes with age-restricted apartments or condominiums.

Other names for retirement communities:

- 55+ communities
- Active adult communities
- Adult lifestyle communities
- Life-lease communities
- Retirement homes
- Senior apartments
- Seniors' housing

Independent retirement living features:

- Apartment-style one- to two-bedroom units in a community setting
- Convenient location near retail shops and recreational activities
- Community features like gardens, pools, golf courses, hair salons, and fitness centers
- Options for housekeeping, meals, laundry, and transportation. One main meal a day is usually offered as part of the cost and other meals are optional at an additional cost, but each unit is equipped for preparing meals
- Transportation for planned excursions

Independent living may be a good choice if the person:

- Needs minor assistance with activities of daily living
- Does not have family or friends that are close by or willing to assist
- Needs a place that does not require a lot of maintenance and upkeep
- Likes the idea of socializing with peers and having activity options nearby

Some seniors do not wish to live exclusively with others their own age, so there are alternatives to an independent living community. I know that my own father was adamant that he would not live with a bunch of old fogies even though, in my opinion, he was one himself. They can consider moving in with a family member or simply moving to a more accessible apartment or condo that is not necessarily age-restricted. The key is being in an area with good access to transportation, services, and social networks.

2. Supportive/Assisted Living

Assisted living is a housing option for adults who are mostly independent but need help with some activities of daily living, including minor help with medications. People in this environment do not require the skilled care provided at a long-term care home. This type of living combines accommodation/housing, hospitality, and/or health services. There are two models of supportive/assisted living accommodations: larger facilities that have many residents, and smaller residential homes that provide similar care to fewer residents in a home-style setting.

Larger residential facilities can be broken down into four levels. Level one ("residential living") is for people who have the least need for support services and who can manage most of their daily tasks. Level two ("lodge living") is for residents who can manage some daily tasks but need assistance with others. Level three ("assisted living") residents require help with many daily tasks, and level four ("enhanced assisted living") residents require help with most/all of their daily tasks.

Other names for supportive/assisted living:

- Residential care
- Board and care
- Congregate care
- Adult care home
- Adult group home
- Alternative care facility
- Sheltered housing
- Independent supportive living
- Retirement care
- Supportive housing

Some assisted living facilities provide apartment-style living with scaled-down kitchens, while others provide rooms. In some, a room may need to be shared. Private rooms may be provided at a higher cost. Most facilities have a group dining area and common areas for social and recreational activities. Other features include:

- Access to visiting or on-staff health care professionals, such as occupational therapists, physical therapists, nurses, and physicians
- Assistance with bathing, dressing, grooming, eating, and mobility

- Health and exercise programs
- Housekeeping and laundry service
- Meal service
- Medication management
- Social and recreational activities
- Transportation to appointments and events

3. Residential Care Homes

Residential care homes are private homes that have been adapted to provide assisted care services for a smaller group of residents, usually no more than 15. These homes provide a more intimate, home-like community atmosphere and offer both short-term and long-term care.

Other names for residential care homes:

- Abbeyfield-style assisted living
- Adult family home
- Adult foster care home
- Family care home
- Care home
- Group home
- Personal care home
- Residential care home services

Residential care homes offer a level of care that varies widely from home to home, but in general, live-in caretakers prepare meals and provide assistance with activities of daily living. Some residential care homes employ or are operated by nurses and can offer care comparable to that in a nursing home, often filling the gap between independent living and nursing homes. There are also residential care homes that specialize in memory care.

Residential care home features:

- Comfortable private or semi-private rooms
- Daily home-cooked meals
- Housekeeping and laundry service
- Medication management

- Social programs and activities
- Transportation to appointments and events

An assisted living facility may be a good choice if:

- More personal care services are required than are feasible at home or in an independent living retirement community.
- Around-the-clock medical care and supervision is not required.

4. Long-term Care / Facility Living

Long-term care / facility living is normally the highest level of care for older adults outside of a hospital. In this type of accommodation, residents receive assistance in activities of daily living and, unlike in other forms of senior housing, a high level of medical care. A licensed physician supervises each resident's care and a nurse or other medical professional is almost always on the premises. Skilled nursing care and medical professionals such as occupational or physical therapists are also available.

Other names for long-term care / facility homes:

- Nursing home
- Auxiliary hospital
- Supportive housing
- Abbeyfield-style assisted living
- Adult family home
- Adult foster care home
- Family care home
- Care home
- Group home
- Personal care home

In addition to medical care, long-term care / facility homes provide residents with a range of services, including:

- Comfortable private or semi-private rooms
- Three nutritious meals per day
- Housekeeping and laundry service
- Exercise and physical therapy programs

- Social programs and activities
- Twenty-four-hour staffing and personal assistance
- Medication management
- Pain management and hospice care

A long-term care facility may be a good choice if a senior has medical and personal care needs that are too great to handle at home or in another facility, perhaps due to a recent hospitalization or a chronic illness, which has gradually worsened, or needs a higher level of care temporarily after a hospitalization, but is expected to be able to return to home or to another facility after a period of time.

If you thought I made your head spin with the descriptions of the various types of dementia, your head is probably ready to explode with all of this information. As if dealing with caring for someone with dementia isn't enough of a strain!? But we need to talk about one more thing, and it's probably what you're most worried about: What are the accommodation options for someone with Alzheimer's or dementia? Are they different than the care provided in any of the facilities described above?

5. Alzheimer's Care / Dementia Care

Seniors with Alzheimer's disease or another form of dementia require special care that is sometimes referred to as "memory care." This care is usually provided in a secure area of an assisted living community or long-term care facility, most often on a dedicated floor or in a designated wing. The secure aspect of memory care communities is intended to prevent residents from wandering off and becoming lost, which is a common and dangerous symptom of Alzheimer's disease and dementia. The security usually takes the form of alarmed exit doors rather than locked exit doors.

Other Names for Alzheimer's care / dementia care:

- Alzheimer's care
- Alzheimer's special care unit
- Memory care
- Alzheimer's care / dementia care services
- Secure care

Alzheimer's care / dementia care features:

- Around-the-clock care
- Comfortable private or semi-private rooms
- Three daily meals
- Housekeeping and laundry service
- Medication management
- Exercise and physical therapy programs
- Structured social programs and activities conducted by staff members specifically trained to care for those with Alzheimer's disease and dementia
- Twenty-four-hour staffing and personal assistance

Placing someone in Alzheimer's care / dementia care is not an easy choice, but at some point it may be necessary to provide a safe and secure environment that has specialized care and staff. Not everyone can afford 24-hour care for an Alzheimer's patient for the extended period of time that it is needed, which is sometime years. Also, a place where the staff is trained in dementia care is an advantage to the person requiring that type of assistance.

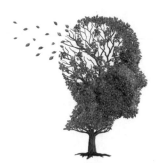

Battle tip: Many different types of living arrangements are available for seniors and each type of accommodation may be referred to by more than one name. Special attention must be paid when moving people with dementia into long-term care as these individuals have unique needs and require a facility designed to meet them.

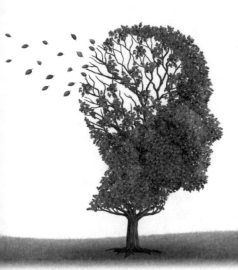

Chapter 6
My Story:
The Long-Term Care
Facility Experience

Making the decision to put a person you are caring for into a long-term facility is undoubtedly one of the most difficult decisions you will have to make. I did not have the information provided in this book when the decision was made for my mother.

One day I discussed the issues of my mother with the staff at the assisted living residence, and very shortly after that I was told that they had found a place for my mother at a long-term care facility. I was encouraged to take this placement, as it was not known when another vacancy would appear. I felt pressured to move quickly and, in hindsight, I think I could have done more research before making this decision. I recommend that anyone faced with this situation take the time to learn all they can about potential long-term care facilities before making a move.

To be fair, the staff were very caring and they did the best job they could. One positive reason to move to this older, long-term care facility was that my mother's doctor was the doctor on call. Mom had been a client of this doctor for many years, and I thought that she would find some comfort and consistency having him visit her there, although I'm not sure she even recognized him. I guess I felt better thinking that she might get a familiar feeling from him. I also had a great deal of confidence in this doctor and knew he would be an advocate for my mother.

The long-term care facility was a very old building, but it was in a very nice area with a lovely deck at the back that overlooked a park-like setting. There were lots of large trees surrounding the building and lovely flowers in the garden. Although that softened the appearance of the building from the outside a bit, it was still a large, square, brick building that looked very institutional.

Inside, the building was painted what can only be described as hospital green, although I am sure it has a more exotic name like "rainforest foliage" or "summer basket green." It was laid out like a typical hospital with a welcome desk at the front entryway.

When you went up to the floor, there was a nursing station just off the elevator and then a hallway leading in two directions to the individual rooms. Most of the residents shared a room due to the high cost of staying in the facility. The rooms had a hospital-type bed for each resident and a curtain that could be pulled between them. There was a bathroom in each room, and you were able to bring a few personal items like a dresser, a small television set, and a comfortable chair or rocker. You could also hang a few personal pictures in the room and bring your own bedspread if you wished. We tried to make my mother's part of her room as cozy and familiar as we could with some favorite ornaments and her own bedspread and familiar chair. Breakfast and lunch were served in a main area beside the nursing station, and the residents were taken down to the main floor for dinner.

My mother cried when we brought her to the long-term care facility. She said that she thought she would never have to move out of the assisted living place that she had thought of as her home, and she could not really understand why she was here. I tried to explain that this would be a better environment for her, but she was very sad. I felt sick to my stomach and thought that perhaps we'd made a grave mistake. I had promised my mother when she was living with me that she would never have to go into a place like this, and I had broken my promise. My mother had never disappointed me but I felt like I had now disappointed her in a major way, and that I had lied to her. I never wanted to lie to her, only to help her. (I would like to stress that you should watch what you promise someone, even if you think they will not remember what you said. It's much easier to tell someone that you will certainly do the best you can to honor their wishes than to make a promise to do or not do something.)

It only made me feel marginally better when the facility called a few hours later to say that she was fitting in well. They told me that they had placed my mother with a wonderful woman for a roommate. It turned out that this lady would indeed be a good friend to my mother.

My mother's roommate had vision and breathing problems but she seemed to be mentally sharp. She acted as a close mentor and friend to my mother. She would help Mom pick out outfits to wear, which seemed strange to me since this lady's vision was quite poor. This roommate always told my mother how wonderful she looked and what a nice figure she had. (Perhaps her eyesight was better than I thought.)

A few incidents at the facility remain a bit of a mystery to me. For example, they always seemed to call to say that my mother needed more underpants. I am not sure why she was losing so many pairs of panties, and I was tempted to go and pull down some pants or pull up some skirts on all of the floors of the long-term care facility to see if other residents were wearing panties with the name "Shirley" on the waistband. I can only assume that she might have been throwing the panties away for some reason, or squirreling them away somewhere.

The staff all loved my mother, as she maintained her pleasant and sweet personality even though her declining memory robbed her of names and the ability to know where she was. I know that many people with dementia get frustrated and angry with what is happening to them. My mother seemed to accept her losses with a calm grace. I know that this acceptance on her part made it much easier for me to bear having her in the long-term care facility. I can only hope that I can be as gracious should I travel this same path in the future. My children harbor this wish on a much deeper level, I am sure.

The nursing staff told me that when the intercom came on with an announcement about bingo or some other activity, Mom would be one of the first people out of her room looking for where to go. I could not believe that my mother was playing bingo because, with all of her accomplishments and the many things she had liked to do in her life, she had hated bingo. I sat with her through one session, and I don't think it was the bingo she was after so much as the chance to be out and with other people. She was randomly stamping the bingo card after every call whether she had the number or not. I did not try to dissuade her from doing so as she seemed to be having fun. I was lucky enough to have a genuine bingo on the card I was playing at the time, and I was rewarded with a prize of five postage stamps. My mother was very happy for me. You would have thought I had won a million dollars!

There was a gentleman at the facility who was only in his forties, but he had some sort of mental disability that required him to be in the home. He spoke no words and only made noises that sounded something like words. This man took a liking to my mother, and they would walk for hours up and down the hallway holding hands. The staff actually had to watch that he did not take her for too many walks each day because she was starting to lose some weight from all the extra activity. I was quite concerned about the attention my mother was receiving from this man. I had heard the rumors and horror stories of sexual escapades between the residents at long-term care facilities, and I voiced my concern to the staff. (Like most people, I'm still not convinced that my parents ever even had sex — well, maybe three times to conceive their three children.) The staff assured me that they kept a close eye on all the residents and nothing of that nature would occur. I gave it some thought and decided it was time for me to grow up: If my mom was getting extra attention, I should be happy that she had some close human contact. If at 86 she could even think about being sexually active, then good for her!

This experience taught me something important. Although people may have forgotten names and people and events, they still crave human contact. The need to feel love and be loved is just as important when you are 86 and have forgotten so much as it is when you are first born and have not yet learned anything. We should not be afraid to touch, hug, hold, and love someone with dementia. It seems like once people are moved into a long-term care facility, every aspect of their lives is decided for them: when to eat, what to wear, when to do an activity, and when to go to bed. I accept and respect that my mother may have craved human touch and that part of her feminine soul found a way to express itself. Dementia can take many things away from someone, but that need for human contact and love is something it cannot seem to steal.

I've read reports that both men and women who develop dementia sometimes make inappropriate comments about sex or act improperly. The articles I have read suggest redirecting the attention of the person to another topic, as these actions may be the result of other things that are bothering them, such as having clothes that are too tight or having to go to the bathroom. If the person is aggressive in these activities, it is wise to consult your physician and not put yourself or others in a vulnerable situation. Intimacy can often be reached through other types of physical contact, such as holding hands or giving a hug. The fundamental need to feel another human's touch always remains.

When I would visit my mom, people would sometimes ask her, "Is this your daughter?" She would look at me for the answer. I always tried to answer cheerfully, "Yes, I am her daughter, and I'm also her favorite child." She always smiled and laughed at this response. I wonder if that was because she was happy to see her daughter, or because she and I both knew that she always liked my oldest brother best.

I used to take my mother out for drives or for lunch on Sundays, and our conversation would go something like this: "Look at those clouds today," Mom would say. And then a few minutes later she would say, "Aren't those clouds beautiful?" Then she might say, "Are you looking at those clouds?" I would assure her that they were the most beautiful clouds ever. If it was a cloud-free day, our conversation was very limited.

One Sunday we went to see the beautiful spring flowers at our city's conservatory. The colors were spectacular and the smells were intoxicating.

When we entered the pavilion, I could hear a drumming sound coming from the center of the building. Mom and I walked over to the sounds and saw a group of people — all ages and sizes — performing what they called a drumming circle. A gentleman who was part of the group asked Mom to join them, and he set this tiny, frail woman down behind a huge drum. I did not know that she would even be able to consider what they wanted from her, but after a while I saw her hand gradually come up to the top of the drum. She began to beat the drum slowly in time with the rest of the group. I was amazed to see her interact with the group and thought this would be my favorite memory of her in her last years. I will remember her as an integral part of the rhythm and circle of life and how she fought and won a little victory over "the big D" that day.

When we left the building where we had shared this experience with several strangers, she turned to me and said, "Wasn't it nice to see all of those people again? We haven't seen them for such a long time, and would you look at those clouds?" Take that, dementia.

I know I was fortunate that my mother did not suffer delusions, depression, or anger like some of the other residents of the long-term care facility. One lady used to cry, "Help! Help! Why won't someone help me?" from a couple doors down from my mother's room. My husband went down to this room one time to see why no one was coming to help. The woman grabbed my husband's arm very tightly and held him there while she told him that they were holding her captive and that he had to help get her out of there. When he said he would go find a nurse, she said they were not real nurses — they were aliens who were holding her captive. The only way he could get her to release her very firm grip was to tell her that he needed to go and get some assistance from outside the room if he was going to help her escape.

My husband came to enjoy the visits to the long-term care facility, even when approached by the "crazy lady" down the hall. He also began to be recognized by one of the male residents, who was often sitting in the front entrance to the home. For months I never saw this very tall and extremely stern-looking inhabitant smile or show any indication that he knew what was going on around him. Suddenly he started to wave and say hello back to my husband when we came in. After that initial contact, he seemed to be waiting for us when we came, and he spent a few minutes talking to my husband each time about the weather or some other subject. He then always waved a friendly goodbye to us when we left.

In a case of this being a small world, the father of one of my best friends from high school was in the same facility. My mother used to play bridge regularly with this friend's mother and knew this couple very well. The friend's mother still lived on her own and would come to visit her husband. She would often stop in and see my mother when she visited. I know that Mom enjoyed these visits, but she no longer remembered her long association with this former bridge-playing friend. If I asked my mom who had been visiting her when I knew her former friend had just left her room, she would just say that a nice lady had been there.

On Friday nights the long-term care facility had what they called Cabaret Nights. After the evening meal, they cleared a dance floor area and played music, and those residents who could, or wanted to, danced. Although my friend's father and my mother had known each other for years, neither seemed to have any recognition or recollection of that. But for some reason they singled each other out as dancing partner on those Friday nights. I like to think that some part of each of their brains acknowledged that this was a friend, and I hope they had some comfort in the human contact they had while dancing. Apparently they only danced with each other. My girlfriend knew this, as did I, but she did not share this information with her mother. She did not want any jealousy to build between the two old bridge friends. Imagine my mother being a homewrecker at the age of 86.

So Mom had one boyfriend that she saw almost every day and a "secret" dance partner on Friday nights. My mother was a popular lady. I believe that these men could sense her inherent beauty. Some things don't diminish, and you often hear stories of people finding someone to care about in long-term care facilities. One lady I know was told that her husband, who had been there for some years, wanted to introduce her to his girlfriend at the facility. He had forgotten that he had a wife, but he had not forgotten love.

I had always joked with my friends that we should have started building our own long-term care facility several years ago so it would be ready when we are. I talked about handsome pool boys and massage therapists that look like Brad Pitt and Tom Cruise. We would have all-white carpets in our rooms, and we would grow our hair out so it would be long and flowing but not so long that it would catch in our wheelchair spokes. The carpet and hair were two fantasies that we could not indulge in while we had young families and messy children and pets. My long-term care facility would be in some exotic locale, preferably with palm trees and an ocean. The long-term care facility in my dreams was one continuous party, full of laughter and fun.

The reality of actually spending a significant amount of time in a real facility severely tarnished that dream. Now I just hope that if I have to go into a long-term care facility, I'll still be aware enough to appreciate any good-looking men working there. I plan to take my feminine soul with me so she can express herself to the end!

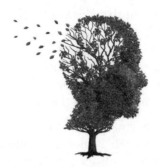

Battle tip: Making the decision to put someone you care about into long-term care is gut-wrenching and difficult. But if you have done your research, you'll be better prepared to take that step with confidence, backed by knowledge, at the time that's right for you and your loved one.

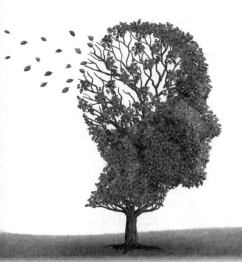

Chapter 7
Choosing and Using a Long-Term Care Facility

Many people still refer to long-term care facilities as nursing homes, but "long-term care facility" is the more politically correct term. I find it interesting that long-term care's acronym (LTC) could also be used for "loving tender care." One can desire that the latter describes what's found in the former.

1. Making the Decision to Take This Step

How do you make the difficult decision to put your family member in a long-term or continuing care center? It's probably one of the most difficult decisions a person who cares about someone with dementia, or any other ailment, must make. You may even deny that it is necessary for a time. I would say that if you're in the process of making this decision, then you must also know in the back of your mind that such a facility may be the best thing for the person: somewhere he or she will be safe and cared for. Starting to think about taking this step is sometimes an indication that you, as the caregiver, are beginning to feel that you can no longer handle this responsibility. As a caregiver, you must realize that if you are suffering from stress-related symptoms, you are not able to provide appropriate care for your loved one. This will undoubtedly be a gut-wrenching and guilt-inducing decision, but it could also be an essential one.

No one wants to deny someone his or her independence and freedom, but there are situations that may make a long-term care facility the best option. For instance, taking this step may keep your loved one from deteriorating further due to poor nutrition or bad eating habits. I know that my mother stashed cupcakes and other food items in her room, wrapped in only a paper napkin, and I shudder to think what germs might have been on those food items when she found them and ate them.

It is not helpful for your loved one to forget to take medications at the right time or to take them too often or not at all. It can also be very dangerous for people with dementia to have access to electrical appliances that could be left on and forgotten. The potential for fire or for the person to injure themselves by electric shock or burns is high. If you cannot be there 24 hours a day, or you cannot afford to have someone else there, then it is difficult to monitor these behaviors.

Of course, there are alternative services that may assist you in dealing with some of these issues, such as Meals on Wheels, where people get well-balanced, nutritious meals delivered to their homes. The daily visit from the person delivering the meals is an added bonus to this service, as it inadvertently provides someone to check in to see if the senior is doing okay.

Many pharmacies offer to put medications in blister packs that make it clear when they are to be taken, and it is easy to see if a dosage has been missed if the pills are still in the slot.

Adult day programs and scheduled programs at seniors' activity centers could provide opportunities for social interaction, to relieve feelings of isolation that sometimes lead to depression. These alternatives may allow your loved one to continue to stay at home for longer. However, if an elderly person has other health or mobility problems, such as broken bones from falls that may have damaged hips or other limbs, or if there has been a problem with getting lost while wandering through the neighborhood, then he or she likely needs long-term care. This is also true if he or she needs oxygen or daily therapy. An inability to handle personal hygiene, such as bathing, or to use the toilet alone is also a clear sign that he or she requires more assistance than someone dropping in occasionally. Any of these things, individually or in combination, indicates that your loved one should be somewhere that provides full-time care and safety.

If you personally have decided that it is time for your loved one to go into a long-term care facility, arrange for a professional evaluation of the situation. A geriatrician or doctor with some geriatric training would be ideal, but if the appropriate specialists are not in your area, you will probably have to rely on others to do the evaluation. Where I live, the healthcare system assigns caseworkers who will conduct an assessment before placing the person you are caring for on a list for a partially government-funded facility. They are trained to do this evaluation, whether they are medical practitioners or social workers. If you wish to pay for private-care options rather than go through the government system, the primary care physician for the person in question is another option. If your physician is not confident in his or her ability to do a proper assessment, ask where you might obtain a second opinion or whether he or she is aware of a facility that does this sort of assessment.

The assessment will determine if the person who needs care can perform "activities for daily living" such as getting out of bed or out of a chair on his or her own. They also check to see if the person can dress without assistance, and will evaluate mobility and balance. There will usually be a test referred to as the "mini-mental state examination" or MMSE. Sometimes also called the Folstein test, this (generally) 30-point questionnaire is used extensively in clinical and research settings to measure cognitive impairment. It can estimate the severity and progression of cognitive impairment and follow an individual's cognitive changes over time, thus effectively documenting an individual's response to treatment. The MMSE aids in diagnosing any type of dementia.

Administration of the test takes between five and ten minutes. It examines numerous functions, including registration; attention and calculation; recall; language; ability to follow simple commands; and orientation. The most noted disadvantages of the MMSE are its lack of sensitivity to mild cognitive impairment and its failure to adequately discriminate between patients with mild Alzheimer's disease and normal patients, but it is a good place to start. If you are at the stage where you feel your loved one may need long-term care, then the MMSE should show indications of mental decline.

On the download kit included with this book you will find a questionnaire called "What Might a Mini-Mental State Exam Be Like?" This is not intended to replace an MMSE, rather, to give you an idea of what to expect.

Talk to others involved with the person being evaluated. What is their opinion on their interactions? Has a neighbor noticed your loved one doing something that seems strange, such as pulling flowers out of flowerbeds instead of weeds or not wearing appropriate clothing for the weather? Have other family members had difficulty with conversations over the phone? Have they come to pick up the person with dementia to find that he or she is not ready or does not seem to remember? Note if your senior has begun missing appointments or often gets lost when driving. All of this should be told to the professional doing the evaluation.

If you believe the time has come for you to put your loved one into a long-term care facility and you have exhausted the possibility of them staying in their current home (either because they need costly 24-hour care or the current caregiver can no longer manage), then you need to start your search for the best home for your loved one.

2. Short-Listing Your Choices

What sorts of considerations need to be made when choosing a new home for your loved one? Before you go to each residence and search for answers to each question posed in Checklist 3 (What to Ask When Choosing a Long-Term Care Facility), begin by shortlisting your choices based on the following (or other important-to-you) considerations.

2.1 Location, location, location

Distance matters when you're looking for a long-term care facility. If you have the luxury of several facilities from which to choose, check out the closest one, where family members or other significant people can visit frequently. A facility that is a five-minute drive away may be best even if you think it is slightly inferior to a home an hour away. The longer drive may seem okay in the summer, but think of those winter days when the days are short and snowstorms can occur. Would you drive an hour each way to see him or her then? Close proximity also makes it easier to check regularly on the quality of care.

2.2 Check the ratio of staff to residents

The number of caregivers is one of the best indicators of good care. An ample supply means staff have time to help your mother out of bed and into her slacks or to nudge her to engage with peers. It means her array of blood pressure and pain medications is closely tracked and she is monitored for side effects, drug interactions, and overmedication. Good turnover data, if available, is a much better indicator of the quality of staffing. It is not unusual for a home to have annual staff turnover of 50 or 100 percent or even higher because of low pay and the job's demanding physical requirements.

2.3 What is their definition of dementia care?

Oftentimes, a facility will tell you it has a special-care unit, which actually means they have a lot of people with dementia and they have a locked unit so those people can't wander off. That's an example of a poor definition of a memory care unit. Good dementia care includes a staffing ratio of five patients to every one staff member, with nurses and aides available all the time, not just during the day. The home should have a positive relationship with local health professionals: GP, community physiotherapist, speech and language therapist, chiropodist, dentist, audiologist, and optician, to name a few. They should also have access to personal care specialists, like hairdressers and massage therapists, who understand how to care for people with dementia. Heading up the dementia care team should be a manager whose door is always open and who is approachable, good at listening, and equally good at making changes where needed.

2.4 Does staff have special training in dementia care? What does that training entail?

You want staff trained in the best ways to address residents with dementia and their unique needs, and who are aware of and sensitive to these needs. This type of care is "person-centered," where the individual needs of the person being cared for are considered. This includes treating the person with compassion, dignity, and respect. If the care center has not embraced the newest type of dementia care being offered, such as the Butterfly Care Homes, described in section 2.5 have, or the newer "village" type of living modules, then check that the staff has had specific training in dealing with dementia. Often people with dementia cannot express themselves well verbally, so staff need to find an effective way to communicate with the residents. Ask how they do this. Also, because dementia care or memory care units do have to deal with residents who wander and may get lost, ask how they keep the residents interested and engaged while remaining in a closed environment.

2.5 Has the facility explored the latest in dementia care?

There are some exciting new changes in the way that facilities can approach responding to people living with dementia. One of the latest models has been recommended by Dr. David Sheard, a world-renowned expert in dementia care. He has developed the Butterfly Care Homes project, where patients' feelings matter more in their care than structure and organization. In Butterfly Care Homes, a wide range of quality of life and quality of service outcomes focus on 12 important points:

1. Employing a house model: Creatively and cost-effectively breaking the care home into domestic-scale, recognizable houses.

2. Creating housekeepers: Transforming outdated ways of working—redefining domestic and catering staff as housekeepers who become the heart of each house.

3. Removing "us" and "them": Clearing away boundaries and barriers that separate us from feeling people's lived experience, and providing an environment that emphasizes — and visibly demonstrates — the quality and value of close relationships.

4. Removing controlling care: Enabling staff to understand how each moment in the day is an opportunity and choice to turn a potentially controlling or neutral task-orientated response into a real, positive, social, and shared connection.

5. Removing central dining rooms: Preventing the "herding" of people from one room to another and creating a positive, engaging, and social occasion where food preparation, visual choices, sensory stimulation, and social connections turn mealtime into a key part of social interaction in the day.

6. Matching: Preventing people from experiencing unnecessary stress by being muddled together when they are at different stages of dementia. Grouping them in "houses" where everyone is at a similar point of experience gives those living there the best chance to thrive and have a sense of well-being while enabling staff to provide specialist skills to these focused groups.

7. Relaxing the routines: Giving the staff team permission to be with people, while fostering teamwork to allow them to still flexibly and discreetly run the home.

8. Filling the place up: Turning the home into an engaging place with loads of opportunities to reminisce, touch, feel, carry

objects, and be engaged in domestic living. This requires an overexaggerated "staging," bringing "stuff" closer to people.

9. Enjoying mealtime experiences: Training staff how to sit and "be with" people, sharing a meal while keeping the conversation going by rehearsing conversation topics, introducing memories, and placing engaging items on the table, in pockets, etc., to talk about.

10. Turning staff into butterflies: Helping staff draw on a wide variety of ways to engage and occupy people in the moment, from wearing "activity belts" (full of objects that start conversations) and connecting with people, to lifting the atmosphere with short minute-by-minute activities.

11. Feelings before behaviors: Providing a set of "recipes" for staff on the meanings behind behaviors. Training staff on approaches that acknowledge that people living with a form of dementia rely less on facts, logic, and reason, and therefore trust feelings more.

12. Measuring well-being: Giving staff practical tools to increase peoples' well-being and decrease ill-being. This involves helping staff see that quality of well-being is the primary indicator of good quality dementia care.

Another new development in dementia care is the concept of creating a village for dementia residents, as was done in 2009 in the tiny village of Hogewey, outside Amsterdam, The Netherlands. An article in *The Atlantic* describes the village:

> Dubbed "Dementia Village" by CNN, Hogewey is a cutting-edge elderly care facility — roughly the size of ten regulation-size football fields — where residents are given the chance to live seemingly normal lives. There are only 152 residents. Like most small villages, it has its own town square, theater, garden, and post office. Unlike typical villages, however, this one has cameras monitoring residents every hour of every day, caretakers posing in street clothes, and only one door in and out of town, all part of a security system designed to keep the community safe. Friends and family are encouraged to visit. Some come every day.
>
> Homes resemble the 1950s, 1970s, and 2000s, accurate down to the tablecloths, because these details help

the residents, who live in groups of six or seven to a house. Residents are cared for by 250 full- and part-time geriatric nurses and specialists, who wander the town and hold a myriad of occupations in the village, like cashiers, grocery store attendees, and post office clerks. Finances are often one of the trickier life skills for dementia or Alzheimer's patients to retain, which is why Hogewey takes money out of the equation—everything is included with the family's payment plan, and no currency is exchanged within the village.

Let us all hope that these newer techniques in dealing with dementia will become the norm in the future for care facilities.

2.6 Ask others

It is always helpful to ask others with family members in the places you are considering if they've been happy with the care being given. Your physician or social worker is also a good resource for information. Check out the websites for the facilities you are considering to see if they have things that you think might interest your parent or loved one. For instance, if the person loves gardening, does the facility have a garden where residents can assist? If your parent's first language is not English, could someone assist with interpretation? Do they offer an art program?

Once you have narrowed down your search to a few facilities you think may be suitable, then go on to the next step.

3. How to Discuss the Move

This can be one of the most gut-wrenching conversations you'll have with the person you are considering for long-term care. Overcome your personal fear of having this discussion by understanding the following:

1. Realize that you didn't cause your loved one's illness or illnesses. He or she will continue to suffer from them whether you are the sole caregiver or there is outside help.

2. Understand that sometimes professional care is necessary for the safety or comfort of your loved one and/or for you to have some life apart from caregiving.

3. Take time to grieve your loss. Being the primary caregiver for a vulnerable person is a huge responsibility. We need to make

decisions about things that seem to have no right or wrong answers. Yet we have to decide. Once we've done so, there will be consequences, whether that means change, or life staying as it is for a time.

4. Understand that you can't live life for other human beings. You can only help them so much. Total control of events isn't in your hands, either. Do your best, and then try to let go.

5. For the most part your loved one will be well cared for, so practice letting go. Do what you can for your family member, and then move forward with your own life. You'll have more to bring to all of your relationships, and that benefits everyone.

Once you have come to personal terms with the decision, you can approach the family member who requires care. It is quite common for people with dementia to have a sense of denial about their problems. This even has a name — anosognosia — a condition where the afflicted person seems unaware of his or her state. It has been estimated that up to 81 percent of dementia patients have this form of denial (Sarah Stevenson, "Anosognosia and Alzheimer's," *A Place for Mom Senior Living Blog*, March 22, 2016). It seems to be the way the brain deals with the problem of losing certain abilities. Our right brain is wired to detect anomalies and new information and incorporate these into our sense of reality, says neuroscientist Dr. V.S. Ramachandran. When something happens to damage that part of the brain — a stroke or dementia, for instance — then "the left brain seeks to maintain continuity of belief, using denial, rationalization, confabulation and other tricks to keep one's mental model of the world intact."

When planning the conversation with your family member going into care, consider the time of day and under which circumstances the person will accept the news best. It is also good to remember the word "ARE." That stands for communicating with the person and not —

A: arguing,

R: rationalizing, or

E: explaining.

A person with dementia cannot understand your points. You are better off to just communicate clearly and decisively. Make statements as if they are facts that cannot be argued.

Choose a time when the person is calm and there aren't a lot of distractions. Consider having a doctor, a home health nurse, or social worker tell the person that he or she needs more care than can be provided at home. The person may more readily listen to a professional. If you think your loved one will not be receptive to this type of conversation, you may have to resort to another method to get him or her to accept the move. You may have to tell the person that this is a temporary move that his or her doctor ordered and that it will be reviewed after a few weeks.

Most likely the person with dementia will be upset by the news. There may be resistance and resentment, and the person may blame you for having to move. But these reactions should not change your mind about the move. You are making the decision with your loved one's interest, quality of care, and life at heart. The person may feel rejected or abandoned. Address these issues. Be patient and reassure your father, for example, about his value, both as a person and as a member of the family. Reassure the person that you love him or her, and that you will visit. Help the person express and handle feelings about the move. Do not argue with his or her feelings, it only makes him or her defend. It is normal for people with dementia to get upset when you bring up such a move, so stay strong and don't take it personally. It is the dementia talking, not your loved one.

4. Make a Personal Visit

If you cannot visit the facility yourself because of time constraints or distance, then try to find someone you trust to make the visit. You will probably have to make an appointment in advance to tour the facility, as staff do not like to disrupt the residents any more than necessary. Take along Checklist 3, and use it as an evaluation tool for the various facilities.

Be ready to use all of your senses, from sight to smell, to profile each home. If you can visit more than once, do so at different times of day and on different days of the week. You may have to be inventive to get in for another look, but you want to have confidence in your choice. On Saturdays and Sundays, for example, the facility may operate with lighter staff, which could compromise residents' care. Mealtimes can be particularly revealing; observe the routine, the quality of the food, and the attention paid to residents who require help.

4.1 Look with "dementia eyes"

When visiting, try not to be swayed by such things as a beautiful lobby or spiral staircases at the entryway, which may say little about the

Checklist 3
WHAT TO ASK WHEN CHOOSING A LONG-TERM CARE FACILITY

Residents

1. Do residents appear happy?
2. Are residents clean?
3. Are residents dressed? (Residents should be in day clothes, as opposed to pajamas.)
4. Are residents alert?
5. Are residents dressed in attire appropriate to the season/temperature?
6. Are residents well groomed (shaven, clean nails, clean clothes)?
7. Are most residents out of their rooms?
8. Are residents lining the hallways, or participating in activities?
9. Are residents' glasses clean?
10. Speak to residents and ask them their opinions of the home.

Policies and Procedures

1. What are the policies and procedures for communicating changes in a resident's condition to family members/substitute decision-makers?
2. Do the home's visiting hours suit your needs?
3. How do family members, or substitute decisions-makers, participate in developing the care plan?
4. How often are residents' teeth brushed?
5. How often are residents bathed?
6. Can a resident choose between a bath or a shower?
7. Who is responsible for labeling personal clothes and belongings?
8. If the facility labels personal belongings, what is the process for doing so?
9. How often are personal clothes laundered?
10. Will the facility accommodate people if they like to sleep in or go to bed late?
11. How do staff communicate with residents who do not speak English?
12. How do staff communicate with residents who are cognitively impaired?
13. How do staff ask non-English-speaking or cognitively impaired residents if they are in pain?
14. Is there a police reference check for each member of staff?
15. Is there a police reference check for each volunteer?
16. What is the home's fall prevention program?
17. What is the home's toileting program?
18. How often will the attending physician see the resident?
19. Will the resident be seen by the physician regularly, or only if there has been a change in the resident's condition?
20. Can a resident keep his or her own physician?
21. What are the policies and procedures for ensuring that personal clothes and belongings are not lost or stolen?
22. What happens if residents' personal belongings or clothes are lost or stolen?
23. Do family members or residents have access to a washer and dryer? If so, is there a fee for using them?
24. If a personal belonging (e.g., personal chair) breaks, who is responsible for the repair?
25. Is cable available in each resident's room?
26. Is each resident able to have a personal telephone?
27. Who is responsible for cleaning wheelchairs and walkers?

28. How often are wheelchairs and walkers cleaned?
29. Are family members allowed to bring pets to visit residents?
30. Does the home have a volunteer program?
31. How many people volunteer at the home?
32. What are the roles and duties of volunteers?
33. What are the policies and procedures for reporting abuse or neglect?
34. What does an abuse investigation entail?
35. What are the policies and procedures for filing a complaint?
36. What is the home's restraint policy?
37. Is the home a restraint-free residence?
38. What are the policies and procedures for handling a resident who is harmful to him/herself or other residents?
39. What is the frequency of care conferences?
40. How are family members, or substitute decision makers, involved in care conferences?
41. Can the resident use naturopathic medicine?
42. What are the policies and procedures for taking a resident out for a day or vacation?
45. Is there a tuck shop? (Available in many assisted living facilities, not necessarily memory care facilities.)
46. If there is a tuck shop, does it have items that would satisfy the person in care?
47. What are the policies and procedures for an outbreak?
48. Does the home arrange for transportation to appointments?
49. Is there a fee for transportation to appointments?
50. Who escorts residents to appointments?

Activities

1. Ask for a copy of the social calendar.
2. Ask for a copy of the activity calendar.
3. Are there activities/social events that would satisfy the person in care?
4. Are there activities/social events on the weekends?
5. Are there activities/social events during the evenings?
6. Are there activities/social events on holidays?
7. Are there outdoor activities?
8. Are there activities for bedridden residents?
9. Can family members participate in activities?
10. Are there activities that take place out of the facility?
11. How do staff encourage residents to participate in activities?
12. Does the staff ensure that activities are customized to residents' interests?
13. If the person in care participates in an outing, is there an additional charge?
14. If the person in care participates in an outing, what is the method of transportation?
15. Can family members participate in outings?
16. If family members participate in activities or outings, is there a fee?

Staff

1. What is the staff-to-resident ratio (personal support worker-to-resident and registered nurse-to-resident) for the day shift?
2. What are the staffing ratios for the evening shift?
3. What are the staffing ratios for night shift?
4. Do staff appear friendly and approachable?

Checklist 3 – Continued

5. Do staff treat residents with respect and dignity?
6. Do staff address the residents by name?
7. Do staff wear name tags?
8. Do staff knock on residents' doors and wait for a response before entering?
9. Does the home have a medical team that includes a cardiologist?
    a. A dentist?
    b. An ophthalmologist?
    c. A podiatrist?
10. If the facility arranges for dentist visits, how often does the dentist visit the home and what is the fee?
11. Has there been a turnover of Personal Support Workers?
    a. Registered staff?
    b. Management?
12. How many staff members are responsible for caring for the person in care?
13. Does the home rotate staff members or try to keep the same staff members caring for the same residents?
14. Is the social worker available to counsel and assist residents?

Programs and Services
1. Does the home have a restorative care program?
2. Does the restorative care program address both physical and cognitive functioning?
3. Does the home have a palliative care program?
4. If so, does the home have an area for family members to spend the night?
5. Is physiotherapy available onsite?
6. What services are included in the regular monthly fees?
7. Does the facility provide speech and language therapy?
8. Does the home provide religious programming?
9. How often do clergy visit the home?
10. Is there a hairdresser onsite?

Safety and Security
1. Are all doors that lead to stairways or exits closed and locked?
2. Does the home have a secure front door?
3. Does the home have a generator in the event of a power failure?
4. Is there an emergency evacuation plan in place?
5. How often does the home practice a mock evacuation?

Food
1. Ask for a copy of the menu.
2. Would the menu appeal to the person in care?
3. Does the home offer choices for each meal?
4. Is the menu posted for all residents to see?
5. Does the food look appealing?
6. Can a family member have a meal with their loved one? If so, is there a fee?
7. Who monitors meal times?
8. If the person in care likes to sleep in, does staff still offer breakfast to the resident?
9. Are different food consistencies available?
10. Are other food choices available if the resident dislikes both alternatives?

11. Does the menu suit the person in care's cultural or religious regulations?
12. Are you pleased with the appearance of the dining room?
13. How long does it take staff to escort all residents to the dining room?
14. How long do residents wait in the dining room before receiving their meal?
15. If a resident is away from the facility during mealtime, will the meal be provided to the resident upon return?
16. Are snacks provided to residents upon request?

Environment
1. Is the facility clean?
2. Is the facility well maintained?
3. Is the noise level acceptable?
4. Are the residents' beds firm?
5. Is there a comfortable easy chair for every resident, bedside?
6. Does every resident's bed have a bedside table?
7. If there is more than one bed in a room, are they separated with a privacy curtain?
8. Are grab bars located beside toilets, baths, and showers?
9. Does the head of a bed elevate?
10. Is there a call bell located beside the bed, toilet, bath, and shower?
11. Does the facility have air conditioning?
12. If the facility is not air-conditioned, what are the policies and procedures for periods of extreme heat?
13. Are mobility devices (e.g., walkers or wheelchairs) available to residents on an as-needed or short-term basis?
14. Are the linens clean and in good condition?
15. How often are rooms cleaned?
16. What does a private room look like?
17. What does a semi-private room look like?
18. What does a basic (ward) room look like?
19. Is there a secure unit for wandering residents?
20. Are hallways clean and well maintained?
21. Are stairwells clean and well maintained?

Inspections and accreditation
1. Ask to read any inspection reports.
2. How many violations are listed on the report?
3. Were any of the violations reissued or repeated from previous reports?

quality of care provided. Try to see the facility as your loved one might. They are looking for a place that is safe and where the quality of care is more important than fancy furniture or decorations.

One good sign is a full parking lot, with visitors being welcomed into the facility to participate in activities and engage with the residents. Are interesting activities going on at the time of your visit, such as music or crafts? If all the residents are parked in front of a TV, then perhaps they are not getting the daily stimulation they need. Don't get me wrong, sometimes television can be a good activity, but certainly not all the time, every day. Do staff seem to enjoy interacting with the residents? Laughter in the hallways among staff and residents is usually a good sign.

4.2 Do the smell test

The unmistakable odor of urine in the facility may suggest that staff-to-patient ratios are not enough to manage the incontinence. This is a primary issue. The facility should want to keep residents dry and comfortable not only because the smell is unpleasant but because urine-soaked bedding or clothing can lead to skin irritations and infections. Catheterization should never be used to manage incontinence, as long-term use invites infection that can be deadly in people with compromised health. Check out the bathrooms available to the residents, both in their rooms and in central areas, to ensure they are clean and accessible. See if the bathrooms have adequate bars and safety devices to keep residents from falling. Ask if there is a regular bathroom schedule that the staff tries to adhere to for the residents. If you can visit early enough in the morning, you may be able to smell if the residents are being attended to during the night to make bathroom visits. A strong urine odor is a good indicator that there is a problem, but a strong antiseptic smell may be a way to cover up poorly managed incontinence.

4.3 Check staffing

Ask for information in a friendly, nonconfrontational manner. Ask questions about the ratio of staff to residents and the facility's turnover rate. Be aware that different regions have different regulations, and there are currently no overarching regulations that long-term care facilities must follow.

High staff turnover is a special challenge for long-term care facilities. Three out of four staff leave every year — that's a new staff person about every three months. Studies show that high turnover rates lead to generally poorer care. It only makes sense that a smaller turnover rate is a good thing. You could also talk to some of the personal care attendants about how often employees seem to come and go.

Even if turnover is low, scheduling can hamper care. Most facilities have a rotating staff schedule, which means the residents see many different faces during a week. The more consistent the contact between your loved one and his or her care attendants, the better they will understand his or her needs and be his or her advocates as well.

Ask what kind of background check the long-term care facility conducts on its staff. Also find out how many of the staff are temporary/part-time or if they are all permanent staff members.

A first impression of an abundant staff level may be misleading. Some staff may be private duty nurses/companions hired by families to supplement the care provided by the home. Ask an administrator or nursing director how many of the apparent staff members you see have been hired privately.

4.4 Find out how they fulfill individual needs

No facility is best for everyone, so look for the facility most tailored to your loved one's needs. An 87-year-old being discharged from a hospital stay for a major medical problem such as pneumonia may need a shorter time in the facility but will require a higher level of nursing care. Any resident with a chronic condition such as diabetes will need management of that condition, so ask how they deal with these types of issues. Does your mother need rehabilitation as she recovers from a broken hip, or has your father had a stroke, which means he now requires speech therapy? Don't accept generalities like "We deal with these types of things all the time." Ask for specifics — the number of hours of rehabilitation care that will be offered — and check with your own health professional to see if what they provide is adequate. If your parent is now unsteady on his feet, ask how they prevent falls. Nighttime trips to the bathroom can be a source of falls, so it's helpful to know what the facility does to try to avoid them.

4.5 Talk to the staff directly

If you can talk to the staff on the floor during your tour, ask them what they like about working at this facility. These are the people your loved one will spend the most time with, so it's good to observe how they interact with the residents and with each other. Do they treat the residents with respect and appear to be interested in their well-being? Ask if they ever use restraints on the residents and, if they do, in what situations? Are staff members out where the residents are and engaging with them or are they separated and talking amongst themselves? Ask as many nurses and aides as you can about how they feel about their workload and how long they've worked at the facility.

4.6 Find out about mealtimes

Poor dietary habits and malnourishment are a real concern for elderly people, whether in a facility or not. If it is not mealtime when your tour is being conducted, drop back in when it is and see if those residents who need assistance to eat their meals are being cared for properly. It can take 30 minutes, or longer, to help such a person eat safely. Do the residents all eat together, or are they separated into smaller groups, or are they getting their meals in their rooms? Hydration is an important part of keeping the elderly nourished, and fresh water should be readily available in all parts of the home. Do the meals look interesting and appetizing? Take a look at the menu for the week to see if there are a variety of items to choose from. Some facilities will encourage family members to join residents for meals, so see if this is an option. That way you can get a first-hand opinion of the type of food being served.

4.7 Look for activities

Are more activities than bingo or TV offered? Can your parent participate in something that he or she has done regularly for years, like an art or dance class? Music can be an important part of people's lives, adding enjoyment and tapping into deep memories not lost to dementia. It can bring participants back to life, enabling them to feel like themselves again and stay more in the present. Can the facility set up personalized music playlists, delivered on iPods and other digital devices?

Excursions outside the facility, such as to a museum or a park, should happen at regular intervals. Many facilities have a large volunteer group to assist in these outside activities. Sometimes students are brought in to do skits or just to interact with the residents. Are live musicians brought in to perform? Special events for the families, such as barbecues or holiday-themed parties, should happen regularly.

4.8 Talk to others

When you encounter a resident or family member during your tour, or outside in the parking lot, tactfully ask him or her the questions that are most important to you and your family member. If most concerned about incontinence, you could ask, "Have you ever had issues with finding your parent in a soiled condition?" If your family member is prone to wandering, ask if that has ever been a problem for his or her loved one and how it is dealt with here. Many facilities have resident or family councils that may be able to offer advice and comfort.

5. Followup after Moving Day: Stay Vigilant

I must stress that you cannot stop paying attention after a loved one has moved in to the chosen facility. You hope and pray that you've done your due diligence and that the facility you've chosen is a good one, but regular followup is strongly encouraged.

5.1 Expect a period of adjustment

The first few weeks are bound to be difficult and it may even take a few months to get a person with dementia through the trauma of the placement. It will undoubtedly be a tough time for the caregiver because you will see this as the beginning of the end and constantly question if you've made the right choice for your family member. If you notice a significant decline or dramatic changes in health after sufficient time has passed for adjustment to the new routine, it may be time to review the situation to ensure that adequate care is being given. Do recognize, however, that once people have been moved into a long-term care facility, they are at that stage of life where they are likely to pass away within 18 to 24 months of being admitted due to normal aging (Chris Orestis, "Life Expectancy Compression: The Impact of Moving into a Long Term Care Facility on Length of Life," lifecarefunding.com, February 12, 2013).

5.2 Monitor medication use

An ongoing concern in long-term care facilities is the use of medications to keep people quiet so they're less of a risk to themselves and others. Besides lessening mental acuity, anything that discourages residents from getting out of bed and being active can have a negative effect. If you have a power of attorney or representation agreement for your family member you can check what drugs the person in care is being given, and investigate the effect of these drugs on the elderly.

5.3 Treat the staff with respect

Feeling guilty about having to admit a family member into a long-term care facility or being distraught and feeling helpless as a loved one's health declines are normal emotions, but there is no reason to take out your emotions on the staff. Getting extremely angry and shouting at staff members will rarely encourage better care for your family member.

The goal is to have these essential caregivers as your partners in obtaining the best care possible on your dad's behalf, especially when you are not around.

Consider the staff as part of your team. As team members, you should have the same goals and everyone should know what those goals and objectives are. Get involved as much as you can. Lighten some of the load on the staff by coming regularly to take your mother for a walk on the grounds or assist in feeding her lunch. By identifying with your continuous and consistent attention, the staff will be encouraged to provide more attention themselves to your loved one.

Share some things of particular interest with the staff members on your team, such as personality quirks or medical highlights about your family member. Work with the staff by bringing in some of your mother's favorite classical music CDs or arrange for a time when she can work in the garden if that is what she loves to do.

Let the staff know that you want to hear about any specific problems they may be having with your family member and look for solutions together. I heard of one resident with dementia who became highly agitated when staff tried to get her to take a shower in the mornings. Her agitation was resolved when her adult daughter found out what was going on and explained that her mother's parents had been killed during the Holocaust. Strangers taking her to the shower had a very specific meaning for her. So the routine was altered: The daughter brought her mother's bathrobe — a familiar, safe reminder of a bathroom routine — and was present several times when her mother showered. The schedule was moved from the morning to later in the day so her mother wasn't groggy and disoriented and, to avoid an unfamiliar face, the same aide provided assistance as often as possible.

5.4 Be aware of changes at the facility

Changes, not necessarily positive, can come suddenly and from unexpected directions. Has there been a change in management or has a source of funding been cut? Perhaps there have been major staff layoffs or a large number of staff quitting. Regularly chatting with staff about future plans or significant changes that occur might help you catch wind of potential problems before they happen.

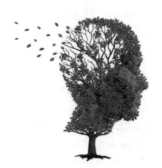

Battle tip: Many things need to be evaluated and questioned prior to choosing a long-term care facility. Follow the points listed in this chapter and always remember to look at the facility through the eyes of a person with dementia.

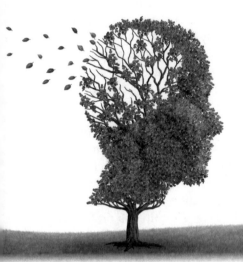

Chapter 8

My Story:
My Mother,
Other Mothers,
My Husband

1. The End for My Mother

When the end comes for a loved one, it is never easy. Sometimes it comes quickly and is a total shock and surprise, and sometimes it comes slowly. When someone you care about has been diminishing before your very eyes for years, you would think that saying goodbye would be easy. But it is never easy to say goodbye to someone you love.

Dementia forces you to say goodbye over a very long period. At first you grieve for the things that the person with dementia has lost: memories and the activities she did that made her happy. You then grieve for what you have lost: your best friend, your companion, your counselor, or your lover. My mother was still with me in that her body was here. I think that, deep inside, her spirit was still there too, but the mother I knew had left some years before she passed. Still, when a loved one dies, no one can prepare you for the loss you feel, even though you tell yourself and anyone else who will listen that it was for the best and you are glad her suffering is over.

The losses began when my mother's lovely roommate disappeared one day. When we inquired, we were told that she had been sent to a hospital due to some respiratory problems. After several weeks we noticed that all of the roommate's clothes and personal items were gone, and the staff seemed to not want to discuss her whereabouts with us.

I was sad because this lady had been a good fit for my mother and Mom seemed even more lost without her. Shortly, another lady was moved into the room but she was completely bedridden and not much company for my mother. Mom did not ask about her former roommate, but I saw how she carefully examined the new lady each time she came in and out of the room, trying to figure out who she was and why she was there.

Mom would often be watching television when I visited, but she would not be watching a show. It seemed like she was watching the "snow" on the screen. "Do you want me to change the channel to something that you like?" I would ask, but she would say that this channel was fine. I think that her fading eyesight probably contributed to her not really caring what was on the television. It was on for the noise, to drown out other sounds, and to make her appear as if she was doing something other than just sitting in her chair.

My mother seemed to lose interest in eating, and I could tell that she was losing weight. It was not uncommon when we went out now for lunch for her to just play with the food on her plate with her fingers. If I tried to feed her she might open her mouth for the first bite but then she'd just shake her head "no" if I tried again. For some time, she'd had difficulty using utensils, but she had been managing to feed herself with her fingers. I asked the nursing staff what was going on, and they said that they had scheduled my mom for some tests at the hospital the following Friday. My mother had not been complaining about anything, but she had just quit eating. Apparently this is quite common in people with Alzheimer's disease; they are unable to articulate that they are suffering from any pain or discomfort.

The long-term care facility took Mom to the hospital by ambulance that Friday, and my husband and I followed in our car. We were sitting in the waiting room when a young technician came out and asked if we were her family. We said that we were.

"I am having trouble doing the ultrasound on your mother," she said. "I cannot get her to lie still and straight. Could you come and help me, please?"

We went into the small room where my mother was curled up in the fetal position on the examining table.

"Please, Mom, you have to stretch out and let her do the ultrasound on your tummy," I said.

My mom tried to straighten out but I could tell that it seemed to be painful for her.

"Please, Mom, let me take your hands and Ron can take your feet so we can hold you still while this nice young girl does her test," I begged.

So I took her hands and held them over her head and my husband took her feet and held them down. She was only making guttural sounds at this point, and it seemed to pain her to lie this way. The technician was trying very hard to be quick as she ran the ultrasound machine over my mother's abdomen. My mother continued to squirm and try to twist away.

"Come on, Mom," I said. "You had three children and have suffered through worse things than this. You can do it. Just try to relax and calm down and they will be finished much quicker than if you struggle. Just look into my eyes and think about something nice. We are here for you and we want to find out what is wrong with you because we want you to get better."

With what I can only describe as the stare of an animal that realizes it is caught in a trap and cannot escape, my mother looked into my eyes. It was all I could do to keep from crying and to tell the technician to stop the stupid test.

"Can she not have some painkillers?" I asked. "This must hurt her."

My husband's voice seemed to soothe her the most. It does have a rich timber and is very comforting in tone. "Come on, Shirley," he crooned. "That's my girl. You are being very brave and I am so impressed with how you are doing."

This seemed to relax my mother enough that they were able to finally get a good — or in this case bad — reading.

They brought my mother a painkiller of some sort, but she seemed unable to swallow it and kept spitting it out. I took another painkiller and crushed it up into a spoonful of ice cream that I bought from a vending machine. She seemed to swallow that, and then they came and gave her a shot of something that put her to sleep.

It was at that ultrasound test that I last saw my mother's eyes open. Although I want to remember the kind, loving eyes of the mother who loved me, I instead see the frightened and wild, trapped-animal eyes that stared out at me during that examination.

The results of the tests were very bad. The cancer that she fought and defeated more than 20 years ago had come back with a vengeance and taken over most of her abdomen. No wonder she no longer wanted to eat.

My discussion with her doctor was very disturbing. He said she had no chance of fighting off this cancer. It would kill her and it was only a matter of time—perhaps days, perhaps weeks—until she died.

"Will she suffer any pain?" I asked him.

He assured me that he would keep her on doses of morphine to keep her comfortable, and I encouraged him to give her as much morphine as he could. I knew that it might shorten her time on Earth, but she had suffered enough and it was time for her body to go.

As a person's body shuts down, it does not need the same nourishment it needed when it was actively living. The body conserves what little energy it has and, as a result, needs less nourishment. In the days (or sometimes weeks) before death, the body seems to exist on nothing, and a non-medical person may wonder how a human can go on so long without any form of food or water. Without knowing this information, I am sure that many people think that the person who is dying is starving.

We sat by my mother's bedside for several hours each day when she got back to the long-term care facility. She indeed seemed to be sleeping comfortably and showing no signs of distress. After spending a lot of time with her one Sunday afternoon, I asked the nurse how much longer my mother could go on like this.

"It is difficult to say," she said kindly. "It could be quick or several days yet. Why don't you go home and get some sleep, and come back later."

We arrived home and about an hour later they called to say that my mother had passed away. We raced back to the long-term care facility and the nurse said that they had brought my mother out to the nursing station so they could watch her. She had taken her last breath without any drama. I was very grateful that she was not alone when she passed away and tried hard not to belittle myself for leaving her. Several of the nurses came up to tell us how much they would miss my mother and that she had been such a kind and polite lady.

That is how I think you can best describe my mother: She was a lady.

I kissed the shell of the body that had been my mother and wished that I could stop feeling overwhelming guilt about not being there when she died. I can rationalize that she did not really know that we were there, but how do you ever know? Perhaps our leaving was a signal for the nurses to give her that final morphine dose and I was responsible for her death? I know that these are all irrational thoughts, but they were the ones that raced through my brain at the time. It is not uncommon to have many thoughts and questions at a time like that.

On the other side of the equation, I was glad that my mother was at peace and that she no longer had to wonder what was going on around her or who all of these strangers in her life were. Her 88 years on this planet were over. I had said my goodbyes to my mother many times over the past years. I know that I lost the essence of her in small increments over time until all that was left was the shell that had once held her vibrant personality. I was surprised at how sad I felt, considering I had wished for her to pass on many times to end her confusion and fear. I guess once death occurs, it strikes you that you will never get the person back. There will be no miracle recovery or sudden reversal of the dementia.

Once that thief has taken those memories, it never gives them back! Once my mother took her last breath and her life was over, any hope of things ever changing for the better were taken away.

I do not think I did very well in this battle. I love the Maya Angelou quote: "I did then what I knew how to do. Now that I know better, I do better." Through this book, I hope to help others know better and perhaps do better.

It is never easy to say goodbye to someone at the end of his or her life. You may make some mistakes as you go through this process and this can lead to regrets in the future. Always remember you did the best you could with the knowledge you had at the time.

2. Friends' Stories: Other Mothers

My friends and I used to discuss the latest accomplishments of our children: Ben's first tooth, Laura's first word, John's first steps, or Erin eating from the dog's dish one day. Now we discuss the latest antics of our ailing parents. I think it is important for people who are going through the same struggles to talk about them with each other. It gives you the feeling that you are not alone, and some of the stories are quite humorous, allowing you to laugh when things are anything but laughable. I do not think that finding the humor in someone's failings is a bad thing. In order to endure the bad things in life, we sometimes have to look at the dark humor or the absurdity of the situation to allow us to process it. Developing a sense of humor is an effective coping skill that can lead to better overall health. You can form a bond with others going through similar situations and it can keep your challenges from overwhelming you. Laughing together can make your very abnormal normal seem better, somehow.

Every time I talk with one of my best friends in Ontario, she has another story about her mother. Her mother suffers from delusions, and although she is taking antipsychotic medication for this, the doses sometimes have to be adjusted. It also seems that if her mother is suffering from some sort of urinary tract infection, her system gets out of alignment and the negative behavior increases.

One time she went to visit her mother and was told by staff at the long-term care facility that her mother had been very distraught. Taking her mother outside for a walk, my friend was able to get her to relax a bit. As they sat on a park bench with my friend holding her mother's hand, her mother shared what was bothering her.

"I think I may be pregnant," she confided.

My friend managed to suppress an outburst of laughter. She had dealt with this type of situation enough times to know that she should not try to convince her mother that she was wrong but that she should rather go along with the fantasy and try to change the subject or divert her mother's attention away from this confession.

"That is very interesting, Mother," my friend said. "I am sure we can find a way to make this go away. Have I told you about the latest things that your grandson is doing? He is starting a fundraiser for a friend of his who has a disease. Isn't that great?" she continued.

"Don't tell your father about this," her mother warned in a conspiratorial whisper, "and we cannot talk about this in that place," she added, as she nodded toward the long-term care facility.

"Mom, I really think we should talk about something else," my friend said, trying to change the subject.

With that her mother burst into tears and grabbed my friend's arm. "Don't you understand what I am trying to tell you? I need your help! It was only the one time and your father doesn't know about it and I don't want him to know. I must find a way to have an abortion. I thought I could count on you for help." She sobbed uncontrollably.

Holding her close in a warm embrace, my friend whispered in her mother's ear. "Why, of course I will help you, Mom. I will call your doctor and we will get the morning-after pill. They have a pill now that you can take and it will take care of any unwanted pregnancy."

"No, no, no! You can't tell my doctor! He will tell your father and it will be a big scandal. You must find another way!" The woman was panicked and her grip grew tighter and tighter on her daughter's arm.

"OK, OK, Mom. Let me go. I will find another way. Now listen to me. Don't you worry about this anymore. I will make discreet inquiries, and I have a friend who is a pharmacist. I am sure that she will help us without any questions being asked. Now, let's go for some ice cream."

With that last comment, her mother got a gleam in her eye and off they went for an ice cream. The matter was not discussed again that afternoon. My friend thought that this would be the end of that conversation; in previous incidents, her mother would forget the delusion and be onto another topic the next day or even five minutes after talking about one of her fantasies.

My friend was astonished the next day when her mother took her aside and, after carefully looking around to see that no one was listening, said, "Did you get the stuff?"

"What stuff?" my friend asked, hoping that her mother was talking about something other than their previous day's conversation. Surely she could not still be speaking about the unplanned pregnancy and believing that she had betrayed her marriage with a one-night stand.

"The stuff to get rid of this baby inside me," she said.

"Oh," my friend thought, "why is she still going on about this?!" She wondered if something had happened to make her mother think she had been unfaithful to her father. Had she had some sort of relations with someone and now her guilt was manifesting itself? Did her mother have an affair decades ago and the memories were just now coming back to her? Was an unwanted pregnancy such a tremendous fear from the past that it was now manifesting itself in this delusion?

While these thoughts whirled in her brain, my friend realized that she had to take the situation one step further. While pretending to rummage through her purse, she transferred some breath mints into a bottle of Tylenol. She then glanced around and said, "Good, there are no nurses around now. Let's go into your room and I will get you a glass of water so you can take two of these pills. They will solve your problem."

She guided her mother into her room and got a glass of water, then watched as her mother downed the two breath mints.

"Are you sure this will work?" her mother asked.

"Absolutely!" my friend said. "I will call you tonight and you can let me know how you feel."

Later that evening my friend called her mother to inquire how she was feeling, sure that the whole incident would be forgotten. She was again surprised when her mother said, "I think they worked, you know, the pills. Please remember not to tell your father."

The next day my friend went to see how her mother was progressing and there was no mention of the previous day's proceedings. It was never discussed again.

In the few years since, my friend's mother no longer remembers being married to her husband of more than 60 years, so she no longer thinks about hiding information from him. At the same time, many things are now hidden from her, such as her memories of her children, where she is, and who she is.

She still, unfortunately, suffers from frightening delusions, which showed themselves when the long-term care facility took residents on a day trip to Niagara Falls. The residents often went on day trips, and my friend's mother seemed to enjoy them. On this particular day, she decided about halfway into the one-hour drive that they were taking her and the other passengers to be killed. She made such a fuss, undoing her seatbelt and trying unsuccessfully to get out of the moving vehicle that they had to pull over on one of the busiest highways in Ontario to try to calm her down. They could not let her out of the vehicle, as she may have run into busy traffic and actually fulfilled the fantasy she was having about this being her last trip. The driver had to phone my friend so she could try to talk her mother down from her delusion over the telephone. This was not a very successful discussion, and in the end the driver had to try to get my friend's mother to take her medication, which she refused to do. This resulted in a long delay on the side of the road until she could be calmed down. Once the crisis was over, they felt it was best to return to the long-term care facility rather than try to continue the outing. My friend was not sure how the other residents felt about having their day trip cancelled, but her mother assured her that they had enjoyed a lovely day out.

Perhaps disappointment caused some of the other residents to be less than kind to my friend's mother over the next few days, or maybe they started to form the pack mentality I saw in the residents when my mother showed signs of weakness or confusion. Or perhaps it was just more of the out-of-sync anxiety that happens to seniors when their routine is changed. My friend soon got another call saying that they would have to put her mother "out" of the home due to her assaulting some other residents.

"What do you mean put her out?" my friend inquired. "You can't just put her out like trash. What are you going to do, place her by the curb?"

The staff said they'd be placing her mom in the hospital until they could get her medications sorted out. This seemed highly unlikely because it was a Friday and the doctors her mother needed to see would not be on call over the weekend.

"Well, did you test her for a urinary tract infection? This seems to be what triggers these events," my friend said angrily. "I will be there as soon as I get off work to resolve this."

When my friend arrived at the long-term care facility, she entered her mother's room to find them finally trying to encourage her mother to give them a urine sample to test for a potential infection. Seconds later, a uniformed police officer arrived asking to speak to her mother. My friend was outraged.

"No, you cannot speak to my mother," she asserted. "You would just upset her. She has no idea why you are here and she cannot communicate properly at the best of times, let alone when she is scared by your presence."

While wondering who would call the police on an old lady in a long-term care facility, the nurses told her that it is standard procedure to call the police following an assault on a resident.

My friend was shocked. They had not told her previously that this was standard procedure, nor had they said they'd called the police. She understood their need to cover their bases, but she was appalled that they did it without warning her and even more outraged that a police officer was invited to the room of a delusional old lady to get a statement.

After sorting out the police officer and the nursing staff, she agreed to take her mother home for the weekend. The staff seemed relieved that her mother would be gone for a while.

Her mother was an angel all weekend and caused no problems, perhaps in part because they'd discovered that she did have a urinary tract infection and they started her on antibiotics. On the Sunday before returning her mother to the facility, her mother sat at the kitchen table while my friend cleared the lunch dishes. She said to her daughter, "You know, I don't know who I am," which about sums up how she felt during those days.

I had felt that I had lost my mother long before she was ever physically gone and here was my friend's mother saying that's how it felt from her own perspective.

My generation has been called the sandwich generation, because we are still caring for children at home while we are caring for our parents. Some may think that being in the middle of a sandwich is great, but it's that part that suffers the most pressure.

It is difficult to transition from being the child to acting as a parent for a mother or father. I think it is important to stress again that their actions do not reflect who they are. People suffering from dementia do not do things deliberately to hurt others' feelings or shock family members. They are simply telling others what is real in their world at the moment, so we should do our best to take nothing personally.

At our coffee table at work, a coworker shared her story. I knew her mother some years before because I had been friends with her oldest son. He was the eldest of six children, and his mother always seemed to be very organized and busy.

As her mother aged, she told us, she had to go into a long-term care facility for problems related to dementia. She had been in an assisted-living arrangement prior to her decline and had many incidents, such as thinking the cleaning staff was taking her items or that the other residents were breaking into her suite. This seems to be a common theme with dementia; it replaces memories with some irrational mistrust.

After getting her mother settled in the facility, they tried to make her room as cheery as possible with portraits of her, her children, and her husband.

One day, while visiting her mother, my coworker noticed her father's picture was not among the photos so she asked why not. Her mother said she'd put it in the bottom drawer of the dresser and that it was not to be brought out because she was angry with him and did not want to see his face.

After asking what her father did to provoke this anger, her mother said, "I have been in this new place for some time and he has not come to visit me once!"

My coworker, astounded, softly said, "Mom, Dad died six years ago. That is why he has not been here. Don't you remember that he died?"

"Oh," her mother said. "If that is the case then you can put him back out on the shelf."

After that, my coworker always checked to see if her or her siblings' pictures were missing before starting a conversation with her mother.

Her mother also developed a deep attachment to a gentleman in the home, and she would often find her mother in her room with this gentleman, either just talking or also holding hands. Was the real reason her mother hid her father's photo so he'd not see her holding hands with someone else? Perhaps the children of people with dementia get their own little dose of paranoia. Maybe it's contagious.

Another friend of mine went to visit her mother in a care facility to take her for lunch. This friend's mother and father had gone on many cruises to exotic places in their retirement years; cruising had been a large part of their life before her mother's move into long-term care. Her mother's eyesight had deteriorated to the point that she was now legally blind, and her dementia was such that her husband could no longer look after her at home.

As my friend guided her mother down the hallway to the cafeteria, her mother warned her that the meal was not likely to be good. "As a matter of fact," her mother said, "this is the worst cruise that I have ever been on and I will not book passage on this ship again." My friend decided not to discourage her mother from thinking she was on a cruise. After all, it's not a bad way to sail into the end of your life.

> Sometimes you have to find the humor in unbearable situations. You may find many other people in your circle of friends who understand what you are going through in the dementia battle. Hearing their stories and sharing your own can help you cope.

3. My Husband's Dementia

I am again attempting to combat the vicious villain dementia. This time it is a battle between dementia, me, and my husband's mind. I hope that we have a bit of a head start this time and can use it to our advantage. Perhaps I know better and can do better.

Let me tell you about my husband.

After more than 25 years of marriage I thought that it had finally happened—my husband, Ron, had quit listening to me altogether. It seemed like his selective hearing was working very well and that the things I told him were not being heard.

I would tell him about an appointment that we had, or some plans for an outing, and he would ask me several times for the details of those arrangements. "Didn't you say we had somewhere that we had to go today?" he'd ask, and I would answer with, "Why, yes. We are to go and pick up the grandchildren and take them to a movie."

"Oh," he would say. "What time and what movie?"

"We talked about this already," I would say. "We are going to the new Disney movie at the theater near us and we thought we would go to the 1:45 showing."

"Great," he'd say, but after a while he would ask, "What movie are we going to?"

"Grr … you don't listen to me! I told you this already. The new Disney movie!" I would say, with a bit of an edge to my voice.

"OK, OK. My memory is not what it used to be. Must be getting old," he would say.

Then he started forgetting important dates and events, like my birthday! Imagine knowing a person for almost 40 years and being married for more than 25 when his or her birthdate suddenly eludes you, even just one day after acknowledging the placement of several pointed hints.

I know that lots of husbands forget these types of dates, but my husband has always been very romantic and considerate of all our special days, so it was totally out of character for him to forget my day. I initially thought it was because he had retired from his job as a cost accounting manager a couple of years before and days and dates did not hold the same meaning for him. Every day was a vacation day for Ron, and he did not have access to a regular calendar or computer to remind him of special days. We did have a calendar on our kitchen counter, but you'd have to go and look deliberately to note the events marked in it. We also have a home computer, but Ron had decided that he did not like using the computer much since he retired. Fair enough, I thought. Still, it was odd.

In 2007, I mentioned Ron's forgetfulness to our family doctor. He seemed to agree with Ron that it was probably just lack of daily exercise for his brain, and that I might need to communicate what was happening a bit more clearly. Ron still did the daily crossword puzzles and seemed to have the answers for even the most difficult questions, so I was sure that his brain was getting exercised. I decided to examine the way that I communicated with him.

I was still working full time and had a busy work schedule as well as after-work social activities. When I looked at how I told Ron about upcoming events and activities, I realized that I'd tell him about everything at once in case I did not get another chance due to my busy schedule. I had my Toastmasters events, and my book club, and dinner outings with my girlfriends that took up lots of my time after work, not to mention the visiting of my children and grandchildren. Because of this, my weekly updates on what I'd scheduled were nothing short of verbal mind dumps, before I'd ask what his plans were and whether he needed me to pick up something at the store. I'm not sure I even paused to take a breath. It was no wonder he stopped listening to me!

I tried to change my ways and mention only what I thought was vital. Then I'd let him ask questions if he wanted more details. It seemed odd to me at first to not share everything I had on my mind with Ron but I realized that I was overloading him with information. Although I'd shared it because I thought it was useful, I decided that all the detail was just cluttering his mind and confusing him.

Over the next several years, I noticed some unusual things, even with the memory problem identified. I think that they were transient ischemic attacks (TIAs) but it is difficult to prove. A TIA is a transient episode of neurologic dysfunction caused by loss of blood flow to parts of the brain that do not cause tissue death. They are sometimes referred to as mini-strokes and can cause some of the same symptoms as a stroke, such as paralysis on one side of the body or sudden weakness or numbness. Dimming or loss of vision, slurred speech, and mental confusion can also occur. Unlike a stroke, the symptoms of a TIA can resolve within a few minutes or within 24 hours, but some permanent brain injury can still occur.

In 2007, Ron had an incident at my son John's 30th birthday party. We had been celebrating on my son's lovely backyard deck on a hot July day when Ron decided to go into the house. He took about two steps and then fell right onto the glass coffee table that was there. He reported having felt like his legs had just collapsed from under him, yet he did not think he'd lost consciousness. He seemed to be okay, but when I took him home to our condo, he was very unsteady on his feet and I had a very difficult time getting him down the long hallway to our door.

Once inside our place, Ron went into the bathroom. I could hear him sobbing.

"Are you all right?" I asked through the door to the bathroom.

"No," he sobbed. "I just want to die."

Alarmed, I opened the bathroom door to find him slumped against the wall. He repeated that he just wanted to die.

"What is wrong? Are you hurting somewhere? Did you bang something when you fell at John's?" I inquired anxiously.

"No, no. I just want to die," he said once more as he slumped to the ground.

I could not get him up and he did not seem to know where he was or what was happening. Frightened, I called 911 and had the paramedics come to the house.

When they got to the condo, they were able to get him on a stretcher and ask him questions. He did not know the date, our address, or our phone number. He did know who I was and he did know his own name and birthdate.

The paramedics decided to take him to Emergency for further testing, which is where we ended up. We were not considered an urgent case and spent a great deal of time in the hallway. We had arrived at about 10:00 at night, and at 2:00 in the morning Ron all of sudden became the "hallway greeter" in the emergency room. He was smiling and waving to everyone who came in and even engaged in conversation with a young man wearing handcuffs who'd been brought in by police officers. As the officers escorted the young man, Ron was asking, "Hi. How are you doing?"

"Stop it," I said. "This is not the place to be Mr. Charming."

After this incident, Ron fell into a deep sleep. I don't know if it was something they put into his intravenous tube or if he was just tired. I spent the next few hours slumped in the chair beside his stretcher. Eventually a doctor came in and administered some tests and told us that we could go home. They said that his heart seemed fine and they were going to book an MRI to see what was going on in Ron's brain. They explained that they could do nothing more and then discharged him. They suggested that perhaps his alcohol consumption, the heat, and the fact that he'd been standing up for a considerable period of time may have all contributed to the fall.

At home, Ron slept for several hours and then woke up quite refreshed, only vaguely remembering the whole incident. He remembered falling at John's, but not much after that. He knew that he'd been in the hospital but thought he'd been in for only a few minutes instead of several hours.

The MRI was done a month later and we saw the doctor for the results. He told us that he did not see anything unusual in the test except for signs of the previous stroke damage in the brain. He suggested that Ron quit drinking to prevent further episodes.

We went home and went on with our lives.

Questions, questions, questions: Over the next several years, my husband's questions increased in frequency, and it seemed like he remembered fewer bits of conversation.

"Do we have any plans today?" he would ask.

"Yes, you have a doctor's appointment," I would answer.

Then two minutes later: "Do we have any plans for today?"

"Yes, I told you that you have a doctor's appointment today."

Then in another two to five minutes: "Do we have anything scheduled for today?"

"Yes, the doctor. Do you remember I told you that? You have an appointment today," I would say.

"What time is my appointment?"

"Two o'clock."

"Is this with my usual doctor? Do I know this doctor?"

"Yes, you know him and it is your usual doctor," I would reassure him.

"OK, what time is the appointment?"

"Two o'clock," I would say.

Then in 15 minutes or so, he would ask, "Is there something we should be doing today?" The question would be repeated until we completed the appointment.

I continued to ask his doctor about the memory lapses and his doctor did regular "mini-mental state" tests on him. The scores were getting lower and lower but medication was not recommended. It would only deter the lapses for a while before they would worsen after taking the meds for a year or more. For this reason, the doctor wanted to wait until the test scores were lower before prescribing anything.

The doctor suggested that because Ron had had a thrombotic stroke a year after our marriage, those areas of the brain that were affected then could now be failing somewhat and causing vascular dementia. A thrombotic stroke is when one of the main arteries to the brain is blocked and the brain is deprived of blood flow for some period. This type of stroke is not necessarily caused by a problem in the heart but is due to a blockage of some sort (cholesterol build-up or fatty deposits cause narrowing and clotting to occur at the narrowed spot). Here is the story of what happened to Ron.

I got a call from the owner of a local convenience store. My husband had stopped in there for cigarettes and was not feeling well and needed me to come and pick him up. The caller said that Ron was dizzy and sick to his stomach and not steady on his feet. I, of course, went to get him. He said that he had a terrible headache and that he just wanted to get home and lie down. I suggested going to the walk-in medical clinic, but he insisted he just wanted to get home.

I got him home and into bed and called our family physician to tell him about Ron's symptoms and ask if there was anything we could do. The doctor thought it might be an inner ear infection, so he prescribed antibiotics. After a couple of days of medication and rest, Ron thought that he was feeling well enough for me to go out for dinner with my mother- and sister-in-law and leave him at home alone. My young children from my first marriage were with their dad, and Ron's teenage son who was living with us at the time was out with friends for the weekend.

I went out for dinner and when I returned it seemed strangely quiet. There were no lights on upstairs, so I assumed that he was downstairs watching television in the rumpus room. I went downstairs and did not see the TV on, nor did I see Ron on the couch. I heard him call "Hi" from the spare bedroom, so I went in to find him on the bed. He had a great deal of trouble talking and he said that one side of his body was completely paralyzed. He had apparently had a dizzy spell while watching TV so he had laid down on the floor and put his legs up on the couch. Then, when he could manage, he had crawled into the bedroom.

What was going on? I called 911 and the paramedics and the firemen arrived shortly thereafter. They loaded Ron into the ambulance and took him to the hospital.

I arrived in my car right behind the ambulance and went into the emergency ward to find Ron. It was a Friday night and it seemed to be an extra busy time for the emergency room staff. I guess they did not consider my husband a priority because he was not bleeding profusely or complaining loudly. I told them about his problem earlier in the week and the potential diagnosis of an inner ear infection. They must have taken this at face value and left Ron waiting in a treatment room littered with bloody gauze from its previous inhabitant. We did not see anyone else for several hours. Finally a doctor came in and tried to make him stand up. When he could not due to the paralysis on his left side, they decided to admit him to the hospital.

They did several tests, but it was not until the angiography test, where they injected a special dye into his blood vessels to track its progress through the brain, that they were able to diagnose the stroke. In Ron's case, they found a congenital narrowing of one of the major blood vessels flowing to his brain, which had caused small clots to form and finally to block enough of the passage to cause the stroke to occur. A stroke had not been immediately diagnosed because Ron's heartbeat was good and he was, at 44, fairly young compared to typical stroke victims. Once the diagnosis was made, they were able to start therapy. He spent some time in the hospital and was transferred to a rehabilitation hospital. They decided against surgical intervention for the blockage because of where it had occurred in the brain. Putting a stint or a shunt in the artery was impossible, so they felt that blood thinners would keep the blood from clotting in this area again.

Ron hated being in the rehabilitation hospital and wanted to come home. They said I could take him home if I continued to bring him in for his daily therapy sessions. We agreed to this and I did not have to be convinced to quit my job for a while to become his driver and care-giver at home.

After several months of exercises on what we affectionately called the killer tomato (inflatable red ball) and the green pea (smaller inflatable ball), he advanced to more difficult tasks. One such task was walking on a trampoline from one end to the therapist who waited to catch him at the other end. Daily flash card readings and bean bag tossing allowed Ron's abilities to slowly return. I think his recovery was partly due to the fact that they picked a cute and buxom therapist for the trampoline therapy. He began to excel at that activity before all others!

Ron was able to walk and talk and he returned to doing all the things he had done before the incident. It was explained to us that smaller blood vessels took over the job of the blood vessels that had expired during the stroke and that they were now the vehicles in which the blood was getting to that part of the brain. To me, it was amazing that we could be like starfish and regenerate new passages to our brain.

We used to joke that his stroke was the golfing god's way of improving his golf swing because he now had to be very careful in how he transferred his weight from one leg to the other to keep from toppling over.

Although his physical abilities returned and he was able to go back to his old job and do it well, he still had some problems. He taught himself the new computer program that they were bringing into the accounting department to prove to himself, and others, that his brain could do it.

One thing that did not return to normal as quickly was his happy and carefree mindset. Ron became suspicious of people and particularly of me. He was sure that I was somehow taking money from him, and every time I was away from the house for any reason, he thought that I was having an affair with someone, or with many! We managed to make it through that difficult period, and we agreed that, although I was undoubtedly totally irresistible to all men, I loved him completely and would never welcome another man's advances.

I am telling this part of the story to point out that the medical system does not always pick up on the symptoms of a stroke in people who either do not show the usual symptoms or are younger than most people who have had strokes. I also found that our family doctor was not particularly in tune with signs of dementia. He seemed quite willing to just let things progress along a certain path and would not pursue other treatments, unless and until I advocated for them.

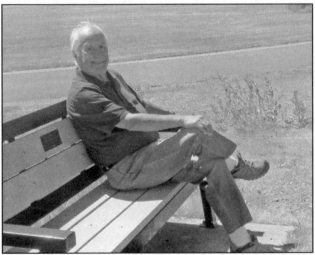

Figure 3: Ron

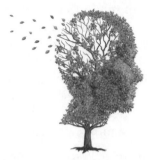

Battle tip: It is natural for spouses to make excuses for their partners and to overlook signs of dementia. As a spouse, you don't want to believe there could be anything wrong, even when you see changes. But you need to acknowledge reality. Make sure you are persistent with your doctor when you see changes that appear to exceed what you would consider normal for your spouse.

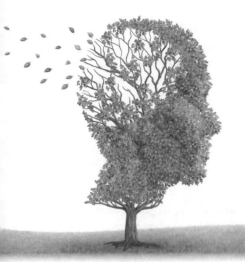

Chapter 9
My Story:
Providing Full-Time
Care Myself

There comes a time when you are caring for a person with dementia or have someone coming in to provide care that you have to decide whether the care is enough. You have to consider the safety of the person if left alone. Is he or she a danger to himself or herself or could he or she wander away alone? Can he or she no longer mask severe memory difficulties?

If the person can no longer be left alone, it's time to decide if you are the right person to give full-time care, or if you should hire people to come in and stay with the person who has dementia, or if it's time for a care home.

If you are in the position where you may have to become a care partner to someone with dementia you should review Chapter 10 for some advice and information on what to expect.

I knew that it was probably time for me to retire from my full-time job on Christmas Eve morning in 2011, when Ron turned towards me in bed and asked the usual morning question: "Do we have any plans for today?"

I answered that we had plans to go to my son Rick's house for the traditional Ukrainian Christmas Meatless Feast that his wife had been preparing for the past 15 years. It was an annual event that had become part of our Christmas tradition.

"Oh," he said. "I just cannot seem to place Rick in my mind. Can you describe him to me?"

My son Rick was not part of Ron and my life together until well into our marriage. When I was 17, I had given up a child for adoption, and it was not until that child was 27 that he contacted me. Ron, of course, had been told about this part of my life before we were married, but neither of us expected this son to contact me. Ron and I had been married about 12 years when I got the letter in the mail. I was thrilled to be reconnected with Rick, and soon after, he became a regular part of our lives. Since that time, Rick and his wife have added two wonderful granddaughters to our family and become an important part of my world.

"You know Rick," I said. "My oldest son; the father of our two oldest beautiful granddaughters. We go to their place every year on Christmas Eve and have the boiled wheat, the borscht, and other Ukrainian dishes."

"No," he said. "I can't place him. Maybe when I see him I will remember."

I retired from my job that January. I needed to spend more time with Ron before he forgot who I was, too!

Once I was at home with Ron full-time, I began to realize just how bad his memory loss had become and I wondered how I had missed some of the signs earlier. Perhaps Ron was just really good at covering things up. I remembered that my mother had a way of being very convincing at times, acting like she knew what was going on when she probably did not.

I realized that I had gradually taken over many tasks that Ron had done previously. For example, Ron decided a couple of years prior to my retirement that he was not comfortable driving anymore. He said he had some cracked vision problems due to his stroke, so I took over all the driving.

I had also been doing all of the banking for a few years, as Ron did not feel comfortable using the computer. I took over making all of the bill payments and handling all electronic correspondence.

Because I was working full-time and Ron did not drive, he no longer interacted with his friends and often said that neither did he need those friendships nor want to continue them. He said that he was quite content to be by himself, doing his crosswords and watching CNN on television.

Ron's memory seemed to take a turn for the worse once I retired. I am not sure if it is because I was with him full-time and interacting much more with him on daily basis that made me notice more, or if he had slipped far more than I had previously thought.

In May 2012, Ron and I were invited to my great aunt's birthday party in Calgary, which I thought would be a good vacation for us. Although Ron did not remember my aunt or any of my cousins, we packed up and drove the three hours to Calgary. We decided to stay in a nice hotel downtown, which was located not too far from where the birthday party was to be held. After checking in and getting ready to go to the dinner, we walked the one and a half blocks to the event. Ron, who was always very social, seemed to be having a good time, and we had a few glasses of wine before dinner was served. Ron said that he was not particularly hungry and he barely touched his meal, but he did continue to take refills on the wine. By the time we left to return to our hotel, I thought that Ron was a little bit drunk but not out of control. I had seen him consume more alcohol than this in the past, so I thought it should not pose a problem. The walk in the evening air would be good for him, I thought.

About half way back to our hotel, Ron stumbled and almost fell. He regained his balance and we continued on, but he said that he felt very weak on his left side. We got to the driveway right in front of the hotel and Ron hung on the newspaper box outside the hotel.

"I feel like I have no strength in my legs," he said.

I encouraged him to try to make it to the hotel so that I could get him into bed. He let go of the newspaper box and collapsed on the street. Several people came rushing by to see if we needed help. Fortunately, an emergency room nurse asked her husband to pull their car over and she asked what had happened. She asked about Ron's previous health issues, so I told her about the stroke he'd had in 1985 and the heart attack that resulted in triple bypass surgery in 1995. She said that she was calling an ambulance and that we should definitely get him to a hospital.

At the hospital, they hooked Ron up to an intravenous drip and started giving him fluids. They tested him and asked him how much he'd had to drink that night. After the results came back, it appeared that this was not a stroke or a heart event but was probably just from drinking too much wine. Ron tried to convince the nurse that this was not the case, but she was adamant that he should quit drinking and, by inference, quit wasting the hospital's time.

After sleeping for a few hours and with his fluid levels topped up, Ron seemed OK enough to return to our hotel. He crawled into bed and fell fast asleep again.

I continue to think that both the event at my son's house some years before and this event were actually mini strokes that cannot be picked up by regular tests. After each of these events, it seemed that his memory issues worsened. I also know that although he did consume alcohol on both those occasions, I had seen him consume much larger quantities in the past that did not result in this type of behavior.

When he awoke later in the day after returning from the hospital, Ron did not remember any of what had occurred, nor did he remember being at the hospital. He actually thought that I might be making some of the story up.

We had a trip booked the next week to fly out to Victoria to celebrate Ron's birthday and our anniversary and to visit the favorite aunt whose birthday we had just celebrated in Calgary. The flight went well and we arrived at our hotel. We did enjoy our stay, although Ron would often ask "Where are we?" and "What are we doing here?" After a few days he started to say "How long are we staying here?" and "Is there some reason we cannot go home?"

Ron did not remember being at this aunt's birthday gathering a few weeks earlier. In fact, he did not remember my aunt at all. She thanked us for coming to her birthday and Ron asked me later what she had been talking about. I told him the story of the fall in Calgary, which he said he could not remember.

Because we were staying in a strange room, the bathroom was not where our bathroom is at home. There were a few times during the night when Ron would get up to go to the bathroom and I would hear the lock on the hallway entrance door to the room being turned. "Don't go out there!" I would yell. "The bathroom is over there, to your right."

I would leave the light on in the bathroom for him, but he seemed programmed to go towards the door that was the entrance to the room. I guess we are lucky that he did not end up wandering the hallways in his pajama bottoms, looking for the bathroom and locking himself out of the room. I know that he would not have known our room number if he wandered down the hallway. That could have been quite interesting and undoubtedly scary for him. It probably would have also scared any other hotel patrons he met.

The trip was fun, though, and we still enjoyed each other's company while on our little adventures. I was worried about him getting lost; but he always stayed close to me, so my fears were calmed.

After our trip, I asked him how he liked Victoria. He said that it was someplace that he had always wanted to visit and that we should go there sometime.

"We were just there for a week," I said.

"Oh, was that Victoria? I thought it was somewhere else," he answered.

About a month after we returned from our trip, Ron made one of his nightly visits to the bathroom. I heard a loud bang and him crying out in pain. I rushed into the bathroom and found him lying on the floor. He was conscious but unable to get himself up, and I certainly could not lift him. He had a lot of wine to drink that night and I was sure that he was just drunk, so I was not too sympathetic. There seemed to be no physical damage to his body and there was no blood, so I brought in a pillow and a blanket. I thought that if he could just sleep it off on the floor for a while, then maybe I could get him up and into bed.

A couple of hours later I heard him calling me. He wanted to try and get up, so I brought in our three-step stool, which enabled him to pull himself up to standing. As I helped him get into our bed, he complained about his side hurting. I could not see swelling or bruising, but he said that it was very painful. I thought he may have cracked a rib if he had fallen on the bathtub next to the toilet. I told him to try to sleep some more and we would see how he felt in the morning.

He did sleep a few more hours, and when he woke he said that his side was still very painful. I called the medical hotline and spoke with a nurse who said I should try and get him into the emergency room to get checked out. Because he was in too much pain to walk to the car,

I called 911. After the episode in Calgary, I was a little hesitant to take him to the hospital again, but he did seem to be in a lot of pain. I was still smarting a bit from the scolding that we had received from the nurse about wasting hospital resources and time.

Once more they did several tests on him and X-rayed his ribs. They found nothing broken so assumed that he must have only bruised his side. Whenever a doctor or nurse asked him questions, I had to answer them — Ron did not know our address or even the details of his fall. After checking with the nurse, I left the hospital for a while to go get him some clothes. But when I came back, he was not where I had left him. Then I saw him in a bed right next to the nurses' station. A nurse then told me that he became quite agitated immediately after I left and tried to remove the heart monitor and the IV and leave the ward. He had been asking where I was. Although they assured him I was coming back, he kept looking for me. "Is he always like this?" the nurse asked me.

"I don't know," I said, "because I usually don't leave him somewhere strange."

The doctor was a very nice fellow who discharged us and said that perhaps Ron should not drink if it affects him like this. I asked if some of these episodes could be TIAs or little mini strokes in the brain, and he said that that was possible but that they were more likely related to his alcohol consumption.

Soon after, we went to see our family doctor, who booked us in to see a neuropsychologist. We went that August for extensive testing and finally got the results: His profile was most notable for a "dense amnesic deficit." That is, he had trouble learning and encoding new information and he rapidly forgot information that had been registered. No amount of semantic cueing or cognition cueing resulted in improved recall. In lay terms, that means that no amount of my hinting could bring memories back for him. He showed slowing on the right-side psychomotor skills and variable performance on visuomotor skills. This meant that he could not do simple tasks easily with his right hand using hand-eye coordination, like putting a ring on a spool. Mild deficits were appreciated on some expressive language tests, visuoperceptual judgment was mildly impaired, and he was unable to complete a map reading test. (Did they know that I'd never seen Ron read a map before the tests?) I guess I was trying to see humor in the situation.

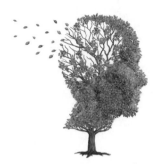

Battle tip: Evaluating when a person's dementia requires you to provide more intensive care can be difficult. Sometimes you don't notice until a particular incident or a string of incidents makes you realize there is a major problem. Try to be honest with yourself about your loved one's behavior so you can identify the need for full-time care as early as possible.

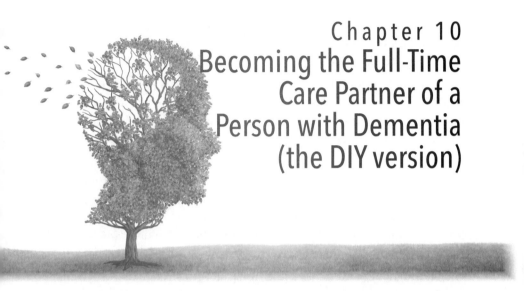

Chapter 10
Becoming the Full-Time Care Partner of a Person with Dementia (the DIY version)

The term "care partner" is the term that many prefer to "caregiver" these days, as it indicates that with an early diagnosis of the disease you are indeed working with the person impacted by dementia to make decisions for what is best for him or her in the future, while he or she is in the early and moderate stages of the disease.

A care partner may not necessarily be a spouse, partner, or immediate family members. It could be a neighbor or a friend who has volunteered to assist in the care of the person with dementia. No matter who the care partner is, he or she should consider the following when developing a plan for care.

It is a difficult challenge for a care partner to determine how much assistance to be giving and when to offer it to the person with dementia in the early stages, as the person may still be primarily independent and resistant to receiving any sort of assistance.

The care partner may have to develop new strategies for supporting the person he or she is assisting and help that person develop new ways to handle tasks without compromising the need for independence.

One of the primary things to consider is the safety of the person with dementia. When considering what I needed to do to make sure that Ron was safe, one of the first things was getting his medication put into pill organizer boxes where each day's dose was in a closed compartment with the day and time on it. This allowed him to only take the pills needed at the required time and not take more than he was supposed to take. I also put a clock in the bathroom that had the date and day of the week displayed so that he had access to that information where his medication was kept.

I cleaned out his closet so he only had essential clothing that was readily accessible when he had to make a choice on what to wear. I still had to cue him sometimes to change a shirt that he might have been wearing for several days but it was easier for him to go to the closet and choose another.

I put a large calendar on the wall where I marked all of our appointments and marked off the days so he knew that the last unmarked day was the current day. I also made an easy-to-read list of important phone numbers and put them by the phone in a prominent place.

I labeled the cupboards and the fridge with what would go where and although I did often find some things in very strange places, I think it did help him find things when he was looking for a particular item.

I removed all the cleaners and chemicals from under the sink and put them on a high shelf in the laundry room so they would not be mistaken for anything edible.

While I was usually available to make all of the meals, if there was a time where I would not be around, I premade something that did not have to be heated on the stove and left it in the refrigerator and put a large note stating where it was and would call at the appropriate time to tell him to eat it.

I took over paying all of the bills and while I would still try to involve him in the process, he did not have access to the bank accounts through his debit card and I took away any credit cards he had in his wallet. I explained this situation to him by saying that we were trying to save for a vacation and that we had to monitor our credit usage and it would be easier if we just had one card (mine).

Ron had decided not to drive some years before, but I understand that it can be a very difficult decision to ask someone with dementia to quit driving. You can enlist your physician to explain that his or her license should be removed for his or her own safety. Some of the red flags indicating it is no longer safe for a person with dementia to drive include involvement in car accidents and minor fender benders, failure to drive at appropriate speed limits, ignoring traffic lights and stop signs, getting lost in familiar places, and near misses.

I made sure that the shower and bath had appropriate safety rails for Ron to hold. I made sure that there was a seat in the shower and appropriate safety mats. I would also start the shower to make sure it was the appropriate temperature before he would step in and later, as his dementia progressed, he did not want to shower alone so I made a point of showering with him.

I tried to make sure that there were clear pathways in the house and there were no tripping obstacles such as loose carpets that could pose a threat.

Since Ron was in denial about having any sort of dementia problems, I avoided using terms like dementia or Alzheimer's to describe his difficulties. We usually said it was his memory issues that we were working to improve with the changes we were making.

As a care partner some of the things that I experienced were:

- **Denial:** I spent a lot of time trying to convince myself that Ron's condition was not as bad as I imagined and that perhaps I was being overly sensitive since I had seen the decline in my mother. In the short term it may have been a healthy coping mechanism to provide time to adjust and accept the problems. However, staying in denial too long can prevent you and the person with the disease from making important decisions about the future.

- **Fear:** My fears about the progression of the disease and the challenges in providing future care could at times be overwhelming and prevent me from focusing on the present.

- **Stress/anxiety:** My uncertainty about what to expect as the disease progressed and how to support the person with the diagnosis definitely led to increased stress.

- **Anger/frustration:** I was angry sometimes, and frustrated to think that the future that we had planned was not going to go the way I expected. I felt a certain level of resentment about how my role as a care partner would impact my life.

- **Grief/depression**: I was also very sad about the whole situation and I was grieving the loss of my partner and my freedom.

I mention these things so that, as a care partner, you can recognize them and perhaps be better prepared to deal with them. You can get a lot of information and support from many places. One of the best things I did was to attend the Family Education Series offered by the Alzheimer's Society. There are many Internet sites and blogs that also offer helpful tips and resources.

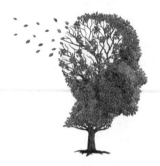

Battle tip: If you have decided that you will be the care partner for a person with dementia, it is a good idea to learn as much as you can about the role and what it will involve. Make safety a priority and work together as partners to find ways to make things work to everyone's best interest.

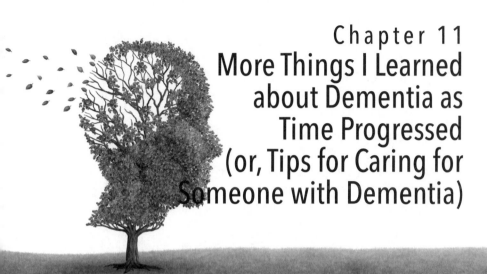

Chapter 11
More Things I Learned about Dementia as Time Progressed (or, Tips for Caring for Someone with Dementia)

1. News and Other Distressing Things for Those with Dementia

A person with dementia can hear the same information over and over again and believe he or she is hearing it for the first time. This can be a good if the information is pleasant, but it's difficult if it's not.

Ron loves to watch the CNN news channel on television. I think he likes that they often repeat the same story over and over again during a day. Although you might think this would help him remember the event, I will tell you a story about watching CNN.

"Where are you, my love?" my husband's voice came from the living room where he was watching CNN.

"I am in the bathroom," I called to him. "I will be right there."

"OK," he said. "Have fun."

"Oh, there you are," he said with relief and surprise when I entered the room. "I was wondering where you were. I thought I lost you."

I sat and watched television with him and we discussed the current events that were on the news show. That day, everything was about the horrible shooting where 20 children were shot by a young man with mental problems. Ron cried over the loss of the children and their beautiful little faces, and said that surely the United States should pass proper gun legislation.

An hour went by and another news program on CNN discussed the same tragedy. My husband said to me as I was fixing our dinner, "Did you hear about this terrible shooting? Twenty little children were shot." He begins to cry softly about the lost little ones. I changed the channel to a cooking show.

The next day I had a lunch engagement with a friend. After explaining that, "Yes, you do know the person but you cannot remember her," and that he could not come along because it was a girls-only lunch, I left the usual note stating where I was going and when I'd be home. He seemed resigned to eating the sandwich I left for him and told me to hurry back.

When I got back he was very agitated. "I didn't know where you were," he said. "I left you a note," I said. "Was that note for today? I thought it was for yesterday. There was terrible news on the TV today. Twenty little children were gunned down." He said those last words with a sob as he sunk onto the couch. I made a mental note to cancel CNN.

We all wish to shield our loved ones from being sad, but I decided not to cancel CNN on our TV because Ron likes to watch the stories, even if they sometimes are distressing for him. He is familiar with the people on that station, and I try to watch it with him and not leave the TV on that channel for hours each day. We talk about the stories, and I always try to make the point that we are so lucky to live where we are safe from some of the terrors that occur in the rest of the world.

I am also trying to get him interested in the home and garden channel, where there is an endless supply of home renovation and decorating shows. We often have good discussions about how we might redecorate our own home after watching these shows.

I encourage him to watch other entertaining shows with me, but sometimes he just prefers listening to his favorite music (Frank Sinatra) rather than watching TV. So many evenings we have Frank Sinatra serenading us while we waltz around the living room. It is amazing the power that music has in our lives. I am sure that long after Ron has forgotten who I am, the tunes of Ol' Blue Eyes will still be familiar to him.

One tip I learned recently is from *Supporting Parents with Alzheimer's* by Tanya Lee Howe (Self-Counsel Press, 2013). If you can, assist the person in your life by creating a Memory Book, where daily activities can be written down, by the person with dementia if possible. This helps the person remember what he or she has done, such as "I had a bath on Monday," and then if he or she is resistant to having another bath it can be pointed out to that it has been several days. You can also use this book to track medication, or as a daily journal to help jog all sorts of memories or simply as a relaxing activity.

You might also create a photo album of the family and a family tree that can be placed in the person's room.

> While we like to shield our loved ones from bad news and keep them from feeling sad, it is not always possible. If a person with dementia likes to watch the news, he or she will see many upsetting things, but if you can talk about it calmly and make him or her feel secure, you can help him or her deal with these stories. You cannot keep a person in a protective bubble, but you can protect your loved one from too many negative stories.

2. Travel with Those with Dementia

I don't think it's possible to decide never to travel with a loved one who has dementia, so you have to take precautions. Make sure others know that your travel companion suffers from dementia and that you would appreciate extra help watching him or her so he or she does not wander off and get lost.

It is necessary to convince the person you're caring for to wear a MedicAlert® Safely Home® or similar device: a necklace, bracelet, or watch. There are many systems to choose from, but the basic premise is the same. If a person is found somewhere and cannot tell the person who finds him or her who they are or where they live, the medical alert system will identify them and notify the contact person indicated on the alert system. This can save several hours of stress for a person with dementia who has wandered off, and do the same for the care partner searching for him or her.

I have also printed out little business cards that I could hand to people when we were dealing with them that said simply, "My husband has dementia. Thank you for understanding." This allowed others to respect his condition and direct any inquiries to me.

When someone with dementia is out of his or her normal environment, he or she can become very frightened and I found it useful to explain several times to Ron that we were going to a particular place and what the reason for the trip was. I would try to show him the invitation to the event or perhaps a picture of the place or person we were going to see, and make statements like "Won't it be fun to see Auntie Anne Marie again?" or "It will be exciting when we get to (wherever) because we have been talking about this trip for such a long time." I did not find it helpful to ask open-ended questions like "What do you want to see most when we arrive in (wherever)?" as those seemed stressful for him to answer. It is not good to overload your dementia travel partner with too much information either, so you must find a balance.

It is a good idea not to plan to do too many activities in one day. Make sure to plan for some rest time. If possible, travel at times when the person with dementia is at his or her best, for example, if he or she gets more anxious in the late afternoon and evening make your travel plans for the morning. It is helpful if you can remain calm yourself and not make any stressful plans such as very short times between airplane connections, etc.

If the person's behavior becomes difficult, do not attempt to physically restrain him or her or try to lead the person away as it may be better to step away and monitor the person while speaking calmly.

A major recent event in our lives was the marriage of my daughter. She decided to have a destination wedding in Mexico in April, and everyone was sent invitations a year in advance. Ron and I discussed all the logistics of the destination wedding, and I showed him pictures of the place where it was to be held.

During the year between announcing the wedding and getting ready to leave for the wedding, there were many incidents where Ron seemed totally confused by what was happening. I was a bit worried about what would happen when we actually made the trip.

Planning for Mexico involved many reminders of what we were doing, where we were going, and why. A few days before leaving, I had the suitcases out, and it was very difficult for Ron to understand that we were not leaving immediately. He seemed quite concerned about what he would wear to the wedding and needed considerable reassurance that he did not need a suit for this wedding, since we had decided that he would wear shorts and a floral shirt. This concept was quite foreign to him, and he kept asking if he had a suit to wear.

I showed him the clothes he'd be taking to the wedding, and we packed the suitcases the night before we were to leave. He got up several times during the night, wanting to know if we were leaving yet and where were we going and why. He also wanted to know if I had packed his suit. It became easier just to say, "Yes, I packed everything we need."

Finally, we were on the airplane to Mexico, and Ron seemed relatively relaxed. We were in a group traveling together to the wedding, and he was good at going along with everyone to get on the bus to the resort.

Once we got to the resort and settled into our room with the beautiful ocean view and warm tropical breezes, he seemed to relax. The first morning, we went down for our buffet breakfast and saw that some of the people who'd journeyed with us to the wedding were already seated. They asked if we wanted to sit with them.

"Do we know them?" Ron asked.

"Yes, they are part of the wedding party," I said.

Some of the people there for the wedding were relatives and long-time friends of mine that Ron no longer remembered knowing. He found it strange that people would come up to him and talk to him using his name, but he was pretty good at discussing the weather or the scenery. Later he would ask who the person was.

On our third day at the resort, Ron asked me in the morning, "Do we live here now?"

"Yes, we moved to Mexico. Don't you love it?" I asked.

"Well, our apartment is a bit small. Where is the kitchen?" he asked.

"I don't cook anymore now that I am retired. We go out to eat all the time," I responded, laughing. "Really, honey, we are on vacation in Mexico for the wedding tomorrow. We are in a hotel room, and we will be going home next Sunday where, sadly, I may have to cook meals again."

"Why do people have weddings that are so much trouble?" he asked.

"You mean why would anyone want to have a beautiful wedding on a beautiful beach with palm trees and sand and the glistening ocean in the background? It is very romantic. That is why, and it is what my daughter and her fiancé want," I said.

The day of the wedding I was quite concerned that Ron would be very confused and not know what to do while I was in my daughter's room helping her get ready. My long-time friend of more than 35 years said that she would get Ron ready and bring him down to the ceremony on time. She knocked on the door and said that I had sent her. She told Ron that he should make sure he had on the outfit that was laid out for him and then she would escort him down to the beach. He did fairly well getting dressed but insisted on his black knee-high socks and dress shoes instead of the sandals we had purchased. But no matter — he was there. My friend said that although he had not seemed to know who she was, he had not resisted being led down to the wedding.

The wedding was beautiful, and Ron enjoyed it and the dinner. When we went to bed that night, he commented on what a beautiful bride the girl had been. He asked me if we knew her.

We went on a sightseeing tour to swim with the turtles the day after the wedding. I left Ron with our beach bag and our camera, suntan oil, and change of clothes, together with our daughter-in-law and our five-year-old grandson on the beach, while my son and the other grandchildren went to get our snorkels, masks, and flippers. We returned to find Ron in a very agitated state. "I lost our bag," he stammered.

"What?! How?!" I exclaimed.

"Well, I had to go to the bathroom, so I took the bag with me for safekeeping and set it down outside the bathroom door. When I came out, it was gone," he said nervously.

"Show me where you went," I demanded. He took me to an outdoor type of bathroom off the beach with a curtain of beads for the doorway and the washing basin outside the curtain.

"I left the bag right here under the basin," he explained.

We went to find security and told them of the loss, and they said they would look around and try to assist us in any way they could. My daughter-in-law told me she was watching her son to keep him from running into the ocean, and when she turned around Ron was gone. He left without saying anything or leaving our bag with the others on the beach.

I must admit that I was upset. Our camera was in that bag, with the wedding pictures on it, and I now had no shoes to wear for the rest of the day; they were also in the bag.

Ron felt very bad, and he could tell I was angry with him. I usually try not to show my anger, but I was obviously not doing a very good job because even my son said to me, "Come on, Mom. Just let it go."

I was trying to let it go, but some part of me did not want to let it go. And Ron could tell that he was in the doghouse; he kept saying he was sorry.

I think I finally came to the conclusion that being angry with him was not helping, when the security guard we'd talked to came up to us with our bag in hand. He had found it at another building a few hundred feet down that Ron must have gone into first, while looking for the bathroom. Everything was there, and it looked like it had not been touched.

I asked the security guard if we could pay him, and he said he was not allowed to accept money for doing his job. So I asked if he could accept a hug, and he said that was OK, so I gave him a big hug.

Ron asked, "Who was that man, and why were you hugging him?"

I said that he had found our bag and that I was very happy, and everything was going to be fine.

Later that day Ron did remember losing the bag, and he mentioned this fact to my sister-in-law. He said that he had lost the bag and that I was angry. She reassured him that it had been found, and he was happy about that but did not remember that part of the story.

It was a reminder to me that getting angry and agitated does not help resolve the issue or make anyone feel good about the situation. My son pointed out to me that Ron was now behaving like my five-year-old grandson, and I should realize that I cannot expect a five-year-old to be responsible for watching something important. I understood that I'd have to adjust my expectations of Ron to be more in line with his current abilities and not expect him to be a rational adult. What's difficult for me to wrap my mind around is that, while my grandson will grow up and become an independent young man, my husband will grow more and more dependent.

Other situations that can cause stress and confusion for a person with dementia is where there is too much chaos or noise. Sometimes gatherings where there are a large number of people and perhaps loud music playing can trigger bad behavior. Large restaurants and concerts could also be a source of distress. It is a good idea to limit exposure to those types of events and try to participate in quieter activities and perhaps only have a few family members over at a time. Go to venues that are smaller and less noisy.

> While we like to shield our loved ones from bad news and keep them from feeling sad, it is not always possible. If a person with dementia likes to watch the news, he or she will see many upsetting things, but if you can talk about it calmly and make him or her feel secure, you can help him or her deal with these stories. You cannot keep a person in a protective bubble, but you can protect your loved one from too many negative stories. There is a joke that says that people with dementia are lucky because they meet new friends every day and everywhere they go is a new experience. On a trip to Mexico with my husband, I learned the truth about that saying. I also learned that I should not expect more of him than I did from my 5-year-old grandson, even though he was 60 years older. They were now on a level playing field.

3. Misplacing Things and Memories

What I once considered unusual behavior is now becoming normal behavior. Things that I could explain away as one-time errors are now regular events. Take note of what is really going on with the person who has dementia to see if his or her problems are increasing.

One of the main worries for all of us is having to leave the person you are caring for alone for a period of time. A major fear is that he or she may wander away from home and get lost or disoriented.

On a daily basis now, things are put in the wrong places: the milk in the cupboard and the cereal in the refrigerator. Ron's keys are often not put back on the peg by the door, and we have to search for them.

I went out one day forgetting to feed our cat his small "morning can" of wet food, so I called Ron and asked him to feed the cat. I told him the can was on the counter and he just had to dump it into the cat's bowl. He said that he saw the can and would do that. When I returned home, I looked in the cat's bowl to see if he had eaten his breakfast and I saw something in the bowl that was very dark and black. When I looked at it carefully, I saw that it was coffee grounds. My husband had poured the contents of the coffee pod containers for our Keurig coffee machine into the bowl. To his credit, they were also sitting in their container on the counter. I was just glad that I did not get a salmon-flavored cup of coffee, and it appeared as if the cat was his usual lazy self in spite of perhaps a few bites of caffeine.

The cat does take advantage of Ron in every way. Whenever my husband goes anywhere within 100 miles of the kitchen, the cat puts on a stellar performance, acting as if he has not had any of his favorite treats for days. Ron, always taken in by this, gives the cat his measured six treats. He can't resist the "A-cat-emy Award" performance. I find it interesting that when Ron remembers little else, he reliably counts out six treats — no more, no less. Perhaps the accountant in him will never die. Needless to say, our cat is getting very pudgy.

On another day, we were looking after my daughter's rather elderly dog while she attended an event. She had brought along some of the dog's special senior care food in a freezer bag so we would have it for the dog's dinner. I was working in our study on the computer when my husband came in and asked what type of snack I had placed on the counter in the freezer bag.

"You didn't eat any of that, did you?" I asked. "That is the dog's food!"

"I did eat some, and it was quite tasty. It had a nice crunch to it."

When I have to be away from Ron overnight, I now use a caregiver service that provides someone to come in and make sure that he has had his dinner and is not too anxious about where I am, and to reassure him that I will be home in a few days. The first time I left Ron for a few days, he called my cell phone several times in the middle of the night to ask where I was and when I was coming home. I had to turn my phone off and make my voice mail message indicate where I was and when I would return so that I could get some sleep and he could hear where I was. I was so anxious to get home that first time, and he was very happy to see me. The next day I still had my suitcase by the bed and he asked me, "Aren't you going somewhere soon?" This lesson taught me that although I was overly anxious and worried about Ron missing me, it seemed like, shortly after my return, he had forgotten I was even gone. This knowledge, that he will likely forget, allows me to take some time for myself when I have to and not feel guilty.

I learned this lesson again when I had a more extended stay away from Ron and could not be in contact by phone. I had inquired about respite stay but decided that it might be too stressful for him to be in a strange environment, so I had the caregivers come in twice a day to make sure he was looked after. Everything seemed to go well and we chatted upon my return about the caregivers and how he managed. He indicated how lonely he was and how glad he was that I was back. The next day we were shopping for groceries and he said, "Aren't you going on a jaunt soon?" I told him that I had gone and that I was back and he said, "Well, that makes me feel so happy! I feel like I just won the lottery." Once again I am sure that he really did miss me while I was gone, but all of that was forgotten very quickly and I was the only one worrying about it.

> My husband's continued strange behavior led to many interesting situations and helped me learn numerous lessons about the disease. One big lesson I learned is that pets will quickly learn to manipulate the situation to their advantage.

4. My Story: Day Program Adventures in Respite and Socializing

Day programs are set up to allow people with dementia to interact with others and so that caregivers can enjoy a time of respite from being constantly on call. I know that I was feeling the stress of being constantly vigilant with Ron and could not find time to do some of the ordinary things I used to do. I felt like I was losing myself and if I was not able to get some relief from caring for Ron my personal health would deteriorate and then I would not be good for either him or me.

Our first attempt to get Ron to enter this type of program was right after we received his diagnosis of vascular dementia. In my eagerness to help, and on the advice of our doctor, we investigated the potential of becoming part of the CHOICE program in our area.

The programs that are developed for seniors all try to keep seniors in their own home environment as long as possible. CHOICE stands for Comprehensive Home Options of Integrated Care Edmonton. We made an appointment for a lovely young healthcare expert to come into our home and interview Ron and me. She asked all kinds of questions and even did a mini-mental test on Ron. When she recommended that Ron go to a day program once or twice a week, I was surprised that he suddenly became very alert and aware of what we were discussing and said that he would absolutely not go into any sort of program like that. He was more articulate and expressive than I had seen him be for some time. The healthcare worker said that if Ron did not sign off on the program then they would not consider him for CHOICE. I found this rather strange, as I certainly did not think that he would have to sign off on the idea. But since I did not have an enduring power of attorney over him at that time, he was considered able to make his own commitments.

His question to the lady interviewing him was, "So, I would go and spend the day with people like me?" She asked him what that meant. He said again, "People like me — with memory problems."

She conceded that there would indeed be people with similar memory problems at these day programs. In response, he insisted that he would certainly not be spending any of his time with people like that. He would have nothing to talk to them about and he would not like interacting with strangers, particularly those with struggles with dementia.

With him suddenly unwilling to participate, even when it was suggested that it was for me to have a rest and not necessarily for him, the idea was dropped. He assured the healthcare person and me that he could look after himself if I wanted to go out; he did not need to be taken care of and I certainly did not have to worry about him when I was out.

The subject was not brought up again until a year later when our doctor asked Ron if he was in any programs yet. He replied that he did not need such a thing.

Our doctor asked him to reconsider and pressed him to think about attending, saying that he thought it would be a good thing for him to do. To my surprise, Ron said that if the doctor thought it was something he should do then he would give it a try. Our doctor put in a referral to a day program.

Within a week, a healthcare worker called me and offered some suitable day programs near us. We gave her our preference and she said she'd get back to us as soon as a spot became available.

A couple of months went by and we received no phone call, so I called the number I had been given and was told that there still must be no room available in any programs. Another couple of months went by and again our doctor asked if Ron was in a day program. I told him the story and he said that he would put in another referral right away.

In fewer than five days from that referral, we received a call from the day care coordinator, who said they had room in a day care program that was very close to our home. I was excited and took Ron over to the seniors' residence where the program was to be held and discussed the program with the coordinator.

The morning we were to go to the program, I had to again convince Ron that his doctor said it would be good for him and that he had agreed to give it a try. He did not want to go, and so I tried to get him to see that it would be a good thing. I was trying my best to make it sound like fun and something he would enjoy. He still did not want to go and I finally had to be really honest with him. "You know I am trying to be the kind and loving and supportive wife that is encouraging you to do things that I think will be good for you, but now I have to tell you that if you don't try this program, I am going to be very angry and it will not be pleasant around this house for some time. So I suggest that you go unless you want to have me be angry at you." He decided to go.

I was not going to stay with him the first Friday, but the woman running the program said that I could. I thought that I would just stay for a short while, but Ron really wanted me to stay the whole day, so I did. The program consisted of an initial social period during which the attendees enjoyed coffee and muffins and then they did some short brain exercises — a word search game and a trivia question game. We then went to exercises where we used small weights and rubber balls to go through a series of movements. The exercises lasted about 20 minutes, and then we went into the movie room, which was set up very nicely with comfortable chairs and a huge screen. A National Geographic film about the Savannah plains was put on, and we got to watch some hungry lions take down a small elephant and eat it for lunch. I thought that turning the lights down very low might be a bit distressing for Ron, and the film, although interesting, was a bit long and not really what I would have shown to anyone just before serving them lunch.

Lunch was served in the room where we had started the day, and it was very nice and fresh. After lunch, we did more brain exercises and then went on a short walk outside since it was such a lovely day. We were then escorted into the large dining room with the other residents of the building to listen to a pair of musicians sing some old-time songs. (I swear that when I get into a seniors' home, I will make sure that they play something more current than songs from the '40s. Hasn't anyone heard of Meat Loaf and *Bat Out of Hell*?)

Several of the residents got up to dance, although perhaps dance is too kind a word. They were moving to the music, which was just as lovely as if they were dancing. They were enjoying the moment. I did get Ron up to do sort of a waltz step for one dance but then apparently he was stuck to his chair for the rest of the session. They served strawberry shortcake to everyone, and the day was over.

The people in this session with Ron covered a few demographics. One lady was 100 years old, but she was very bright and she seemed to enjoy the whole day. Then there was a gentleman in his 70s who also seemed to be enjoying the day and was very good at the trivia. I think that he perhaps had had a stroke, as he showed some symptoms to suggest as much, but he did not seem slow mentally. Then there was a lady who had been a seamstress for her whole life; she had a sweet face and a wonderful smile. She had some paralysis on her right side but was very engaging. Another gentleman seemed to have a good time repeating everything he was given to read, and I was told that he had been a Supreme Court judge in his earlier life but was now pretty lost. He did thank the woman who served him his lunch and said that he thought everything was lovely, so his social graces still seemed to be there, but he could not really answer a question that was put to him directly. Another man was a former RCMP officer who said he'd also worked for CSIS, the Canadian Security Intelligence Service. He seemed to be the youngest of the group and he was very social and talkative. You would think he had no problems, but he did tend to need direction as to which way to go for certain parts of the program. He told me that his daughter dropped him off and picked him up from the program each day. I don't know if he lived with her, but he no longer had his own driver's license.

A former schoolteacher also tried to keep everyone in line, particularly during the question-and-answer, trivia parts of the day. She did not like it if people spoke out of turn, for example, and said that no one would have gotten away with that in her class.

All in all, I thought it was an interesting experience, but it was rather boring for me and I think for Ron too. When we got home from the day program, I asked him what he had liked or disliked about it. He just said, "Liked or disliked about what?"

"The day program we were just at", I said. "Where we just spent the day with all those people doing word searches, exercises, and dancing."

"Oh. I don't remember being anywhere," he said.

The next Friday I again had to convince Ron to go, and he certainly did not remember being there before, but after some coaxing I got him dressed and we set off for our second experience at the day program. I stayed for the first half hour or so and then, when they left to do exercises, I told him that I would be back to get him later and I left. Well, I thought to myself, that was not so bad. Since I had a whole day in front of me, I decided to go for a pedicure. I was nicely in the pedicure chair with my feet soaking when my cell phone rang. It was the day care coordinator. She said that Ron was quite upset that I was not there and that he wanted to leave. I spoke to Ron on the phone and told him that I would be there as soon as I could get there, but it would be about 45 minutes. He said that he wanted to leave right that moment, so I apologized to the lady preparing to work on my feet and booked an appointment for myself and Ron for later that day.

When I got back to the program, Ron was waiting in the lobby with the coordinator and he seemed quite agitated. After we got home, I asked him what he did not like and why he had called me. He said that he did not know but that he just did not like being there. Of course, by the time we went to get our pedicures that afternoon he did not remember being at the program in the morning.

Our third Friday came, and again, over much protest, we went. He only agreed after I promised that I would stay and that we would leave before lunch. I had discussed this with the coordinator, who thought it might be a good idea to have him come for short days at first. I took my book and tried to stay out of the way for most of the day, but I was within sight of Ron so he seemed to be okay. When we left, he said that he really did not like this idea of me not participating.

The next Friday came and, although he could not remember any of the previous Fridays, he had the sense that he did not want to go where I was trying to get him to go. He absolutely refused to go and did not even care when I said I would be angry at him for not going. He was not going even if I said that I would stay the whole time. I was thinking about one of the people in my care partner support group who told me that his wife was so attached to him that when he left her at a day program and she saw a car that she thought was his, she ran out and banged on the car window to be let in. I decided that we would not try the program that week; perhaps we would have a better shot in one more week when he might be more agreeable. The next week came and he seemed even more intractable. I discussed it with the coordinator, and she said that they did not have enough people to try and watch Ron all the time; if he did not want to participate it would be difficult for him and the others. So we stopped going and I decided to wait six months, when I might be able to convince him to try again. It was not relaxing for me to know he was stressed out somewhere on the days I was supposed to be enjoying time off.

I started hiring private companion care to come into our home when I felt I needed to escape for a period of time. I researched several agencies that provide that care and chose one that I had a good interview with and had the same regular companion come. I interviewed the companion who was an older man who seemed to be a good fit with Ron. Ron seemed to consider that this person was a family friend that just happened to stop by when I had to go out without him.

Some people are fortunate to have other family members, or neighbors, or friends, who would consider coming in to provide a couple of hours relief for the care partner. It is important to ask for help. Others might not realize that you need some time off unless they are told.

> Caregivers need respite care. One of the ways they can get a few hours to do other things is to enroll the person they are caring for into a day program. These programs can provide interactive and safe care for a person with dementia, but it is not always easy to get them to participate. If the day program is not an option it is important to get regular respite in another way, either through private organizations or soliciting your family and friends for some time away.

"If at first you do not succeed, try, try again" is a well-worn phrase that could apply to me, Ron, and the day program. Or perhaps the famous saying attributed to Albert Einstein — "Insanity is doing the same thing over and over again and expecting different results" — is more germane in this case.

Sure enough, six months went by and one of the people I go to a support group with told me that her husband was now in a day program at a different facility than the one we tried, and that she was quite pleased with it. Her husband seemed to like this program even though he had not liked previous programs. I hoped that Ron would somehow recognize this gentleman from our support group sessions and that this would make him want to attend the program.

I contacted the program facilitator, who said that she had room for Ron. She mentioned that the livelier group came on Mondays and

Wednesdays and that the gentleman from our support group attended on those days.

I eagerly took Ron to the next Monday session, dropping him off at 9:30 in the morning and picking him up at 2:30. He seemed to be in a good mood and said that he liked the day and had enjoyed this visit. Hurrah! On the Wednesday, he did not remember the Monday visit and questioned me all the way there about where we were going and why. I left him at the program as before, but this time when I came to pick him up he was sitting by himself in an easy chair away from the rest of the group. The coordinator told me that he had begun to look for me around lunchtime and did not want to participate anymore; he just wanted to wait for me.

My hope, that he would somehow recognize the gentleman we knew, was short lived; although they did speak to each other during the day, they showed no sign of recognition. At a special dinner arranged by the day program, we sat at a table with my friend from the support group and her husband and, although they were sociable, it was as if neither had ever seen the other before.

After that first Wednesday, a few warning bells were ringing, but I decided that I had to try and keep him going. The next Monday he asked where we were going and I told him that we were going to the day program. He asked, "What's the day program and why do I have to go?"

Once again I answered him with the facts that his doctor thought it was good for him to go and to interact with others. It took a lot of talking to get him to attend the next few sessions and I was exhausted by the time I got him to the program.

I started to pick him up from the program earlier so that he would be the first to leave. This was the coordinator's suggestion, because she had noticed that Ron became very anxious if someone else left before I'd come to collect Ron. He would pace around, waiting for me to show up.

When I did pick him up, he would always ask me the same questions. "Did you get everything from our room?" or "Do we have everything that we came with? I feel like we are forgetting something."

I would assure him that we had not stayed at the facility overnight but had arrived there in the morning from our home.

"Is home a long way to drive from here?" he would ask.

"No, we are just five minutes from home," I would answer him.

"Really, where are we? Did we move?" he would ask.

As the weeks went by, he found excuses not to come with me when I said it was time to go to the program. He could not remember going, but he felt very sure that he did not want to go. I would sometimes not tell him where we were going, and when we arrived at the day program facility, he would look at me and say, "Don't I know this place? I don't want to be here."

I thought it was pretty amazing that he did not remember being there but had a sense of not wanting to be there. Very interesting and I am sure it would make a good case study into dementia for someone.

We reduced his visits to one day, the day when the young children from the child daycare program that operated next door came in to sing. Ron loves to see children so I thought this would make him willing to attend.

For a short while he did enjoy seeing the children at the program, but then he started to separate himself from the others and wait for me to return. This took a staff member from the program away from the others to make sure Ron did not leave the building.

As the weeks went by, I was exhausted from trying to get Ron to the program, and the staff at the program were exhausted trying to keep him there. The coordinator and I agreed that it would be best if we discharged him from the program. I would try to get a caregiver to come into our home to stay with Ron while I went out to do my errands, and that would give me some respite.

Everything came to a head when I told the program coordinator that I had an upcoming weekend trip planned. I said I would have private caregivers come in twice a day to make sure that Ron had lunch and dinner and took his medications in the evening, as I had done before. She jumped up and said, "You cannot leave him alone at any time now!"

She immediately phoned the case worker assigned to us through the healthcare system and informed him that I needed 24-hour care for my husband for the weekend and that he should get in touch with me immediately. She really scared me and obviously got things moving because they came out that afternoon to assess Ron and his needs.

I booked private 24-hour care for Ron that weekend because the healthcare system could not react that quickly to a request for assistance unless there was some sort of health emergency. (The fact that I just about dropped dead from fright and shock did not count.)

At first I was quite annoyed at the healthcare worker's response, but then I had to realize that she was in a much better position than I was to assess Ron and his needs. I spoke at length with her and she did indeed open my eyes to some of his behaviors.

Since that time I have been able to receive two afternoons a week for my personal respite care from our healthcare system. At first I felt quite guilty about taking this help since I was still thinking that I could, and perhaps that I should, be doing it all. Perhaps there were people with greater needs than mine who could use this type of care.

I had to realize that I was an emotional wreck. I could not take care of Ron the rest of the time if I did not get those critical breaks.

I discuss this further in Chapter 12, section 4., Self-Care. I was suffering from many of the symptoms of burnout but was ignoring them because I thought Ron's needs were greater. That is a mistake for any caregiver; just like in a plane, it is critical that you put on the oxygen mask before assisting others who are more vulnerable.

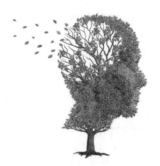

Battle tip: I was unable to let go of the idea that Ron might not fit into a scheduled program and tried a different approach. Unfortunately, I found that he had become used to having me as his sole caregiver and was unable to assimilate into any program where I had to leave him. This situation is very draining on caregivers and finding some method of getting respite care is necessary.

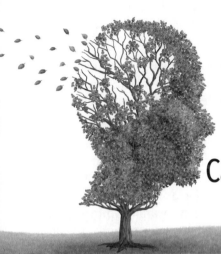

Chapter 12
What to Expect when Caring for Someone with Dementia: Taking Care of the Caregiver/Care Partner

1. Respite

As previously mentioned, the person who is providing the primary care for a person with dementia requires some form of escape and respite in order to recharge and re-energize so that he or she can continue his or her role without damaging his or her own physical or mental health. Sometimes you just need to get away for a doctor's appointment on your own, or to get a haircut.

Respite care can be provided at home by a friend, other family member, volunteer, or paid service, or in a care setting, such as adult day care or residential facility.

In-home care services offer a range of options including:

- Companion services to the individual with companionship and supervised activities

- Personal care or home health aide services to provide assistance with bathing, dressing, toileting, and exercising

- Homemaker or maid services to help with laundry, shopping, and preparing meals
- Skilled care services to help with medication and other medical services

Adult day centers offer a place where the person with Alzheimer's can be with others in a safe environment. Staff leads planned activities, such as music and art programs. Transportation and meals are often provided.

Residential facilities may offer the option for an overnight stay, or a stay for a few days or a few weeks. Overnight care allows caregivers to take an extended break or vacation while the person with dementia stays in a supervised, safe environment. The cost for these services varies and is usually not covered by insurance or Medicare.

Contact your local Alzheimer's organization to get a list of respite providers and ask them if they could provide any information or assistance regarding funding for care in your area. Some insurance plans will cover the costs of respite care so call your insurance provider as well. There are usually seniors' organizations in your area that would also have information on this subject. The Internet can also be a good place to search for assistance.

2. What to Expect Emotionally

In reviewing how I handled my mother's dementia versus my husband's dementia, I realized that the caregiver's emotional experience can be very different depending on who they are caring for. The situations I went through with my mother and my husband were similar but my reactions to each were quite different.

I was extremely sad when my mother was slipping into the world of dementia, yet there was a certain amount of acceptance. After all, my mother was old and you expect these things to happen. Shifting from the role of daughter to that of caregiver was difficult because I had always counted on her to take care of me. But, it was a necessary transition and seemed natural.

The mothering I received from Mom allowed me to do my best to mother her in the same way when she needed it. I knew what made her happy and what upset her. This allowed me to focus on pleasant things to help minimize her confusion and discomfort.

Even though I sometimes felt I had let her down — that I could have done more for her, could even perhaps have kept her at home longer or should have visited more when she went into long-term care — I eventually came to terms with the guilt and accepted that my mom had the best care possible.

The mother/daughter bond remained strong and, although I felt the mother I remembered had slipped away years prior to her actual death, I still loved this woman who had once been such an influential part of my life. I didn't have any negative feelings toward her nor did I dwell on what our relationship could have been had she not ended up with dementia.

With Ron, the situation is somewhat different, even a bit convoluted. There is the same sadness, but some of it is due to unrealized expectations and dreams I had about how our life would be in our golden years. I certainly don't have the same level of acceptance as I had with my mother, and going from wife to caregiver has been a more difficult transition. This shift in responsibilities is anything but natural.

The challenge of having my husband absent mentally and present physically has been difficult. While I always felt I was still my mother's daughter, am I still a wife if my husband doesn't know me? The person I depended on to be my support and sounding board can no longer occupy that role.

When Ron was still at home, I often felt I was living with a stranger — someone who would do and say unfamiliar things. Suddenly, I had to make all the day-to-day decisions. I even had to choose his meal when we went out to eat. I often wanted to shout, "Can't you make one little decision for a change?" I knew he couldn't and that dementia was responsible for robbing him of this ability, but part of me was frustrated. I was much more frustrated with Ron than I was with my mother.

I wanted to love the man who had been my husband for so many years but he wasn't really there anymore. To shift from loving him as a romantic partner to offering him the kind of love a parent has for a child — for that is what our relationship became — was almost impossible. Like countless others, Ron and I had vowed we'd stay together in sickness and in health, for as long as we both shall live, and so naturally I felt responsible for his care. I had to come to terms with the fact that no longer looking after him in our home might be a breach of our wedding vows. I struggled with that idea for some time. Ultimately, I decided that our vows had not stated that one person must totally sacrifice mental and physical health for the well-being of the other. If you had to vow that up front, I don't think there would be many marriages.

The other major difference between dealing with my mother's dementia and dealing with Ron's is that I was not expected to sleep with my mother. With Ron, the issue of sex had to be dealt with.

It is difficult to feel romantic about someone who has become a virtual stranger. But dementia did not seem to diminish Ron's ardor for me. He, if anything, seemed more insistent on having marital relations. I often felt he did not really care, or know, that it was me, his wife of many years, he was having sex with. It seemed that I could just as easily be a stranger that he paid for sex. (This was worse because I was not getting paid!)

For me to feel romantic and in the mood, I like to feel the intimacy of shared thoughts and desires. I like my husband to do the little things he knows I appreciate, such as loading the dishwasher after a meal or giving me a foot rub in the evening. Grand gestures like buying me a dozen roses or a gift aren't required, but I like to know that I am seen and valued/appreciated for who I am and for all that we've shared together. Someone asking me "Do we live here?" or "Which way is the bedroom?" does not inspire that romance. Once we lost our intimate connection, I could not feel amorous towards Ron.

Ron was always a jealous sort of person and often thought that every man on the planet found me irresistible. While this can be flattering, it can also be annoying. I was constantly forced to deny that others had a romantic interest in me or that I had a romantic interest in anyone else. Jealousy intensified for Ron as he progressed through the stages of dementia. He actually began to think I had a millionaire boyfriend waiting for me every time I was going out. I must admit, I sometimes wished the millionaire boyfriend existed!

I developed a rather ingenious way of thwarting sexual advances. If Ron was feeling particularly passionate first thing in the morning, I would tell him, "Oh, honey, that would be great but you really wore me out last night. You were such a tiger!" Of course, he could not remember what had happened the previous night, so he would feel quite proud that he'd been such a stud.

If he wanted to be intimate in the evening prior to us going to bed, I would tell him I had a few emails to answer and then would be more than excited to come to bed. I said I needed to get the task done so I could focus on him. I would tuck him into bed with the promise of coming in soon and then wait for the sound of snoring before retiring. Mean and manipulative? Or clever and cunning? I'm still not sure how I feel about having behaved that way, but it was the best thing I could do for myself at the time.

Some people in my Alzheimer's support group say they still enjoy sex with their partners, and I applaud them. In my case, it just did not feel right. In truth, it almost felt like incest, since I often felt more like a mother to Ron than a wife.

As mentioned previously, I think a lot of my feelings towards Ron are tinged with a sense of loss and unfairness. I imagine that many people go through this same sense of loss when their partners have a terminal disease of any kind. But I sometimes feel that couples going through a battle with cancer or some other illness can pull together, make the disease their common enemy, and fight it as a couple. It's different with dementia. The person with the disease often doesn't realize he or she is ill and can't fight with you against it. I often feel that I am fighting this alone — and going through the battle for someone who does not appreciate or understand what I'm experiencing. At the same time, it sometimes seems like I am actually fighting Ron because he often says there is no problem. He argues with me about doing things that will keep him safe and give me more peace of mind, such as having someone stay with him if I have to go out.

Although it is terrible if your spouse passes away from cancer, heart disease, or other ailments, at least you have the certainty of death at the end. Friends, family, and coworkers surround the surviving spouse and offer support and encouragement. I have not seen this same outpouring of love for people who have been caregivers to someone with dementia year after year. To the caregiver, it may seem like his or her partner died many years ago and yet he or she lacks support and encouragement because, technically, the loved one is still living. I felt grief many times over while caring for my husband. I have suffered a loss but not a specific loss. You cannot say "My husband was lost to dementia on February 2, 2001," when he is standing next to you. You suffer over and over again with each change in the person as the disease progresses.

There are, of course, those short moments of clarity when Ron is himself again. I almost find these more difficult. Although these times are to be celebrated and enjoyed, having Ron there for a moment or two makes it harder for me when he is once more lost to dementia. I often think, "Oh there he is, welcome back! They must have been wrong with the diagnosis." I guess some part of me would like to believe this is not really happening.

Don't ignore the emotional toll that dealing with this disease takes on you. Talk to a health care professional if you are beginning to feel overwhelmed. There are also many organizations that offer assistance for the care partner such as the Alzheimer's Organization in your area. There are usually support groups that you can attend with, or without, your partner, and your doctor should be able to assist you in finding a group. There are usually a number of organizations that you can research on the Internet to find an appropriate fit for your situation or to find an online support group that you could join. One of the most important things to remember is that it is OK to ask for help and support.

> There is a vast difference between caring for a parent or other relative with dementia and caring for your spouse. The emotions associated with losing your partner to dementia can be more intense and harder to accept, and the physical aspects of your relationship may change. Remember that there is help available for you.

3. What Dementia Has Taught Me

This terrible disease has taught me some very important things about myself and about life. I realize that I must live every moment in the moment and enjoy each thing that comes along. After all, I may forget these things in the future and I want to make sure that, at the particular instant that something wonderful is happening, I chose to cherish it.

I have learned that it is not enough to think that you are a patient person; you have to put that patience into practice every day. You must realize that the person with dementia is not saying or doing anything to antagonize you on purpose. He or she truly does not remember asking you something 100 times or telling you the same story over and over. How can you be angry or impatient with someone who has no malice or ill intent?

I have learned that self-care is a very important part of being a care partner for someone struggling with dementia. In fact, I feel that it is so important that I have devoted section 4. of this chapter to addressing that need.

The role of shifting from the daughter to the mothering role that occurred for me with my mother's dementia was a difficult one. Part of me felt that my mother had abandoned me but I knew that it was not her fault and although I loved her dearly, I was a bit angry with her. She was the person that I always called on to give me advice when I was in a difficult situation and now I could not call on her about this problem.

I have found out that it is lonely living with someone you love with whom you have lost that memory connection, whether it is your parent or your husband. It is very difficult to repeat over and over again who the important people in your life are and who family members are. The shared joys of the past are gone; but on the positive side of that same coin, the shared angers and hurts are also gone. Each day you get to begin a new relationship with someone who loves you and vice versa. It is important to remember that the person you love is still in there somewhere and that we all crave the feeling of being loved and important to someone. When a person has dementia, many of the senses are diminished or changed, but the sense of touch is still an important one. I find that often all that is needed is a hug, or holding the person's hand to make him or her feel secure.

I learned from my mother that although she did not remember her children and did not know the people around her, that a person can still be peaceful and calm and not take her frustrations out on others. My mother maintained her sense of calm and her polite demeanor all through her illness. I hope that I have that ability built into my DNA from her.

My mother was still able to smile and laugh even when she was in places that she must have found very scary. I learned to love and admire her in a different way. I appreciated the inner beauty that remained until her final breaths. I hope that I have learned those lessons from her and that I will be able to exude those same characteristics in my senior years. Oh wait, I am in my senior years now. I will wish for that behavior in my much more senior years.

I have learned never to start a conversation with my husband by saying "Remember when … ?" because he simply does not remember. It is interesting to note how often that type of conversation occurs between partners. You want to talk about something in the present but it obviously relates to something in the past that was important, so you start by trying to establish the link between the two things. I found it is better just to tell him the past occurrence. My conversation may go something like, "Honey, we went to that cute bed and breakfast in Montreal a few years ago and this sign on this bed and breakfast reminds me of that place where we had such a nice time. It was called the Petite Prince and this place is called the King's Castle. They are both worthy of royalty, I guess."

I also now include details about my friends or family prior to us being involved with them. For example, when I am going to meet my friend of over 30 years for lunch, I tell Ron, "I am going out to lunch today with Elly. She is my friend that used to be my neighbor on the acreage. Her daughter and mine were born just a few weeks apart." The most important part of this conversation would be "I am leaving at 11:30 and I will return by 1:30." I leave a note with the same information on it and my cell phone number as well. My cell phone number is also on a piece of paper under the telephone. I schedule these lunch dates when I have a caregiver coming into the home for the few hours I am away.

Although I do try to flesh out details about things, I make sure I do not overload Ron with too much information. I try to make sure that my sentences are clear and concise. This is not a normal way for me to speak, as I love to make a long story out of everything.

When Ron has an idea about something that has not happened or is wrong, I try not to challenge his statements, as that usually makes him aggravated. I try to change the subject or just gloss over the statement. Sometimes it is a question such as, "What happened to those people that were just here visiting?" when we had no visitors. I say something like, "Oh, you must have been thinking of the other day when Laura was here. There has not been anyone here today visiting; although it would be nice to have a visitor, wouldn't it?" If I were to say "you are wrong, there was no one here," or "you are crazy and seeing things. No one has been here all night," then he would get argumentative and upset.

Sometimes he gets an idea into his head that something is about to happen, like he is sure that we are going to the grocery store that day. It does not seem to matter how many times I tell him that we are not going anywhere and the grocery store is not happening today, he will continually ask when we are leaving to go to the store. I try to mark it down on the calendar and say that we are going to the store on Wednesday, and it is only Monday so we have two more days to wait, but that does not seem to change the idea in his mind. It is curious to me that he can create new facts in his mind that his brain hangs onto and does not shake and yet he cannot remember something I just told him. The brain is a very strange and interesting machine.

One of the best descriptions I have heard about communication and memory centers for people with dementia came from the Alzheimer's Society in Edmonton, Alberta. It says that your brain has a central repository for communication. A request comes in from the outside for information, such as me asking "What did you have for lunch today?" This request for information goes along the road to the central control area, which directs the courier truck to travel along the road to the short-term memory section of the brain to retrieve the information, which is just stacked up loosely without a lot of organization. But there are many roadblocks along the way, and the retrieval vehicle has to dodge around those blocks. It gets delayed in retrieving the information and sometimes cannot get to it at all. If the retrieval vehicle does get something from the short-term memory, it has an equally challenging time coming back to the central communication system and then transferring that information to another vehicle to deliver the verbal response to the response center. This vehicle also has roadblocks along the way that may cause the final answer to the question (if there is one) to be incorrect. The roadway system to the longer-term memory may have a better maintenance crew who keeps those pathways a bit clearer so that information is more readily retrieved, and that long-term memory section has the memories secured in better filing cabinets that are more organized and readily accessed. See Figure 4.

> Dementia has taught me many things, and some lessons were harder to learn than others. The main lesson is to try to live in the moment. This is good for all us. And remember: For people with dementia, the moment is all they have.

4. Self-Care

One thing that everyone stresses is the importance of self-care during the time of crisis when caring for a partner or family member who has an illness. Again, I liken it to putting the oxygen mask on your own face before attempting to assist others. If you are burned out and unable to function, the person you are caring for will not get the care that is required.

The stress of caring for someone with dementia can lead to emotional, physical, and mental exhaustion. It is mandatory to recognize the

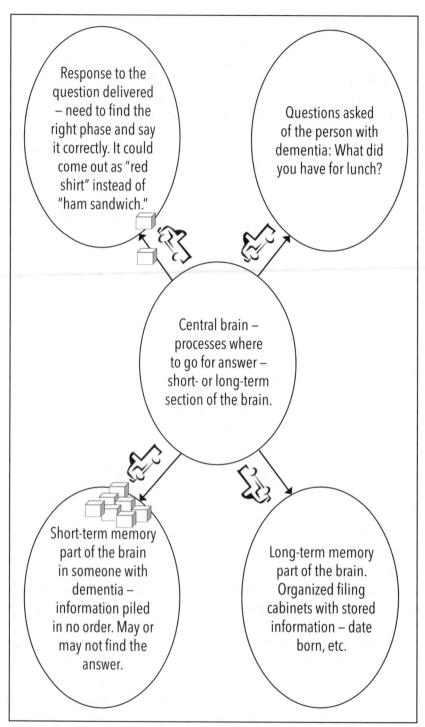

Figure 4

signs of burnout and to take steps to keep yourself healthy. Sometimes the caregiver gets so wrapped up in doing things for the care partner that he or she neglects to find balance in his or her own life. Where others would see an abnormal balance in your life or that you are overwhelmed with what you are doing, it's become your new normal and you have to take a step back and evaluate your situation.

Caregivers have a higher incidence of suffering depression and abusing alcohol or drugs, and they have a higher rate of chronic illness than people of the same age who are not caregivers. It is not selfish to take care of yourself — it is necessary!

Please consider some of these symptoms as possible warning signs of stress and burnout:

- **Cognitive symptoms**: memory problems, inability to concentrate, poor judgment, negative thoughts, anxiety, and constant worrying.
- **Emotional symptoms**: moodiness, irritability, short temper, agitation, inability to relax, feelings of being overwhelmed, a sense of loneliness and isolation, depression, or general unhappiness.
- **Physical symptoms**: aches and pains, diarrhea or constipation, nausea, dizziness, rapid heartbeat, loss of sex drive, frequent colds.
- **Behavioral symptoms**: eating disorders; sleeping disorders; withdrawing from others; procrastinating or neglecting responsibilities; using alcohol, drugs, or cigarettes to relax; developing nervous habits like nail biting or pacing.

It is important to acknowledge the feelings you are having. Perhaps they are feelings of sadness or loss. I know I am very sad to have lost the connection I once had with my husband and that we can no longer share the little inside jokes we once laughed at. The past 30 years of our marriage seem to have disappeared for him and I mourn that loss, both for him and for me. I thought that we would spend our old age together sitting in rocking chairs on the porch, laughing and enjoying each other's company, or perhaps we would spend our golden years traveling to exotic places. I did not think that he would forget our life together and eventually forget me too. I know that when you get married you state "for better or for worse ... in sickness and in health," but I don't think anyone really believes that something like dementia will happen to them.

There is often a period of grief with dementia. Just as there is when you lose a person you are caring for to a death such as are caused by heart attack, with dementia, you grieve as the person you are caring for is still alive. Dementia is a fatal, progressive, and degenerative disease that destroys brain cells, and you must soon come to grips with the fact that this person will never be the same person you once knew. You may grieve the loss of the person you knew or the plans and dreams that you made together for the future; the loss of the life that person once lived; and, in the case of a partner, the loss of a confidant and someone with whom to plan and share your dreams. These are definitely things to grieve. As a caregiver, it is important for you to recognize that the person you are caring for may also be going through a phase of grieving for who they were. The loss you feel is sometimes referred to as ambiguous loss because closure is not possible and your grief cannot be fully resolved while the person with dementia is still alive. It is important to reach out for support and to find ways to deal with your grief. Ultimately, you want to develop a new way of accepting and connecting with the person.

You may also experience feelings of frustration and anger at having to continually answer the same questions and assist your care partner with daily activities that he or she can no longer do alone. Frustration often arises from trying to change an uncontrollable circumstance. I sometimes equate dealing with someone with dementia to having a three-year-old constantly at your side, asking the same questions again and again and wondering where you are all of the time. Just as you would treat a three-year-old who needs your attention with kindness, I hope, that is what you must do with a loved one with dementia.

Recognizing that what you are dealing with is an uncontrollable circumstance leaves you with the only choice available to you, and that is to control how you react to the circumstance. You have the power and control to choose how to respond. I constantly have to remind myself that my husband is not doing these things to annoy me; he cannot help it, and I must try as calmly as I can to respond to whatever is occurring.

If you feel you have made poor choices in how you responded to situations in the past, then you may also feel a great deal of guilt about those choices. Or you may feel guilty when you go out and have a good time with friends or take time for yourself because you think that your care partner cannot enjoy this with you. You may even feel guilty that you no longer feel the same way about your care partner as you used to. Go easy on yourself and try to forgive yourself. No one is perfect, and you can be expected to sometimes react in ways that you had never thought possible.

Another feeling that is often expressed by caregivers is resentment. "Why me?" is a common question. Perhaps you feel that other family members are not sharing the load the way you would expect them to. Why don't your siblings, children, or whoever you think should be assisting you offer to do more? After everything we have done for them, why don't they return the favor? Sometimes you have to ask for what you need from others. If you are busy doing everything yourself, many people will just assume that you are doing it all because you want to and do not need any assistance. Do not be afraid to ask for help.

All I can say is that it is OK to acknowledge your feelings and, as Dr. Phil says, realize that "you cannot change what you don't acknowledge." Recognize that these are natural, normal feelings for a caregiver. You cannot be expected to be a smiling angel all of the time, but you must learn to recognize the warning signals of stress and take action. This may include consulting a professional counselor to help you work through your feelings. Others may find a regular meditation practice helpful for putting things back into perspective. People who have a spiritual connection can use it to find comfort and strength.

Some people find that support groups are an effective way to discuss feelings with others who are going through similar circumstances and can offer suggestions or solutions to problems and issues. Check for such groups in your vicinity. You will find that many of them have options where you can bring a care partner with you. Your local Alzheimer Society is a good place to start.

Do not give up regular contact with your family and friends. It sometimes seems easier to decline offers to go out, but it is important to maintain those relationships. Do not isolate yourself. If you have to ask someone for help while you attend a family birthday or a luncheon with friends, then do it. Perhaps you have to pay for an outside caregiver to come in for a short time while you go out. The price you pay for that service will be more than gained in the fresh perspective you will have after a few pleasant hours out.

One of the most important things that you can do is avoid neglecting your own health by skipping meals or continually eating unbalanced meals, not exercising, or getting reduced hours of sleep each night. It's also important to remember to not neglect your own dental and doctor appointments just because you spend so much time taking your care partner to theirs.

Make arrangements for regular respite care for your care partner so that you can go away for a period of time. Taking a holiday from your regular routine, even if that week is spent just sitting somewhere quiet where you can read or write in a journal or listen to your favorite music without interruption, can recharge your batteries. If you cannot take a few days or weeks off, you can still give your mind a five-minute vacation break by following a simple plan. Just find a spot where you can shut out everything else and put your mind to work imagining you are watching a beautiful sunset on a beach. Also, try to imagine hearing soothing music playing. Even better would be to do this exercise with the music you love playing in the background and having a picture of a favorite vacation spot. By allowing your mind to travel to a beautiful locale for five minutes and relax to some favorite tunes, you can feel like you've had a refreshing break from your daily tasks. You could do this mind exercise more than once a day, too!

Some interesting things have been written about a group of care-givers who were taught to use a regular meditation practice. Several recorded studies showed positive results in providing some relief from the stress of taking care of a person with dementia. So if you can learn to build a daily meditation practice into your life, it could be beneficial.

It is important to set realistic goals for yourself both in terms of what you can do and what you can accomplish for the person in care. Set realistic short-term goals for what you can achieve each day. Perhaps you will not be able to get all of the laundry done that day or clean out the fridge. Let things go that can be done another day if you find that the current day gets too full. It is a good idea to set long-term goals as well and be brutally honest with yourself about what these goals might be, even if they seem unpleasant now. You may have to set a goal of putting your partner or family member in a long-term care facility at some point, and it is good to acknowledge that goal and realize that it is a potentially positive eventuality. Preparing for this as you would prepare to achieve other goals will reduce the stress and self-doubt that you may feel.

One thing that I try to keep in mind is that it helps to retain a sense of humor about the situation if you can. You may think that there is nothing amusing about this disease, but if you can find something to laugh about, it will dispel anxiety, reduce feelings of aggression, and push depression aside. A study done by the Mayo Clinic offers some interesting findings about laughter. A good laugh can actually induce physical changes to your body because it stimulates your organs by causing you to take in greater volumes of oxygen-rich air and increasing the endorphins that are released by your brain. It can relieve your stress response and the tension you are feeling, and leave you more relaxed.

Most important of all is to have compassion for yourself. Offer yourself the same care and understanding that you are giving to the person you are caring for. Stop having negative thoughts about yourself and how you are handling the situation. Do not indulge in negative self-talk. Our feelings and behaviors are largely influenced by the way we talk to ourselves about the situation. Try to reframe the situation in a way that puts the most positive spin on it. Realize that you are doing the best that you can do, and cut yourself some slack.

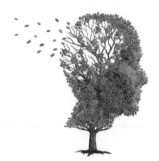

Battle tip: You cannot look after anyone else if you have depleted your own resources. It is not selfish to take care of yourself; it is necessary. Learn to recognize the symptoms that will tell you it's time to start and maintain a program of self-care.

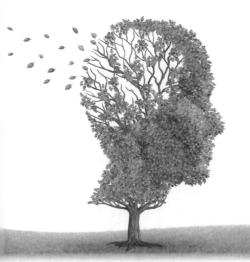

Chapter 13
What I'm Doing about Dementia Moving forward (and What You Can Do, Too)

One thing I am doing about dementia is writing this book, so that I can share my experiences to date with anyone who might care to read it. I hope to encourage and inspire others. I have made it a focus of my life to read as much as I can about this disease and my purpose in writing was to condense the information into a manageable format. I will donate a portion of the profits from this book to the Alzheimer Society.

I am involved with the Alzheimer Society in my area and have talked to second-year medical students about what it is like to be a care partner for someone who has dementia: the challenges, and the perks.

I have participated in a study that is looking at the stigma that remains for those struggling with dementia. I hope that my research and experience will contribute so we can try to develop a better strategy for dealing with this terrible disease, by caregivers and all of society in general.

I do public speaking engagements to senior groups and to anyone who would like me to talk about my experiences.

I have held fundraisers to provide financial support to the Alzheimer Society for research.

I have tried to stay up to date with new studies related to dementia and evaluate if they might be applicable to my husband.

I tell people to make sure that they have their legal and financial paperwork in order. While it may be a difficult conversation to have with someone, it is important to get the proper documentation completed. Documents such as:

- **Will:** a legal document by which a person expresses his or her wishes as to how his or her property is to be distributed at their death, and names one or more persons, the executor(s), to manage the estate until its final distribution.

- **Personal directive:** Sometimes called a living will, health care directive, advance directive, or representation agreement, it is a document which outlines end-of-life wishes, but it's broader. A personal directive can be about all health-care decisions, where you live, the activities you take part in, etc.

- **Power of attorney:** A power of attorney is a legal document that you sign to give one person, or more than one person, the authority to manage your money and property on your behalf.

  Among other requirements, you must be mentally capable at the time you sign any type of power of attorney for it to be valid. In general, to be mentally capable means that you are able to understand and appreciate financial and legal decisions and understand the consequences of making these decisions. However, the legal definition of mental capacity will vary based on the laws in each province or state.

  A general power of attorney is a legal document that can give your attorney authority over all or some of your finances and property. It allows your attorney to manage your finances and property on your behalf only while you are mentally capable of managing your own affairs. It ends if you become mentally incapable of managing your own affairs.

  A general power of attorney can be specific or limited, which can give authority to your attorney for a limited task (e.g., sell a house) or give them authority for a specific period of time. The power of attorney can start as soon as you sign it, or it can start on a specific date that you write in the document.

An enduring or continuing power of attorney is a legal document that lets your attorney continue acting for you if you become mentally incapable of managing your finances and property. It can also give your attorney authority over all or some of your finances and property. An enduring or continuing power of attorney can take effect as soon as you sign it. In some cases, it is possible to have the power of attorney come into effect only when you become mentally incapable, if this was specified in the document.

You can find information about these documents either from a lawyer or from other reputable resources. Self-Counsel Press offers books and online kits that you can use to make these documents yourself, where legal to do so. A call to your local seniors' groups such as AARP (American Association of Retired Persons) or CARP (Canadian Association of Retired Persons) will guide you to the assistance you may need get these documents completed.

Given the number of people who currently have dementia and how quickly that number is growing, I'm also asking those reading this book to take it upon yourself to do something. What can you do? It can be as simple as raising your own awareness of the growing problem of dementia in our society. Or you could take a more active role and raise funding for research into a potential cure for this affliction. It's also important to talk to your family and friends about the symptoms of dementia and what you have learned. Discuss what you would like to have happen to you if you get diagnosed with dementia.

Make sure you have the legal documents mentioned above in place. Self-Counsel Press publishes books and kits on making wills, living wills, powers of attorney, and more: visit self-counsel.com.

If you know a care partner for someone with dementia you could find ways to support them through such things as assisting them in creating a Memory Book, where daily activities can be written down, by the person with dementia if possible. This helps the person remember what he or she has done, such as "I had a bath on Monday," and then if he or she is resistant to having another bath it can be pointed out that it has been several days. This comes from a book called *Supporting Parents with Alzheimer's* by Tanya Lee Howe (Self-Counsel Press, 2013). Help the care partner create a photo album of the family and a family tree so that the person with dementia can have it in their room and look at it.

1. What Others Are Doing

In 2012, Seth Rogen and his wife Lauren (along with some amazing friends), created Hilarity for Charity. They later established the Hilarity for Charity Fund as part of the Alzheimer's Association, through which monies raised are directed to help families struggling with Alzheimer's care, increase support groups nationwide in the US, and fund cutting edge research. Since its inception, Hilarity for Charity has raised more than $6.5 million to support these efforts.

Olivia Newton-John, Beth Nielsen Chapman, and Amy Sky created *LIV ON*, an album to Aid & Comfort Those Experiencing Grief & Loss While Using the Power of Music To Heal.

Glen Campbell: I'll Be Me is a 2014 American documentary film about country music singer Glen Campbell. Glen and his family decided to share their journey with this disease with the public.

Rita Hayworth Gala: Princess Yasmin Aga Khan began this event in honor of her mother, actress Rita Hayworth, who died as a result of Alzheimer's. Under Princess Yasmin Aga Khan's leadership, the 2016 event raised nearly $2 million, and a grand total of over $70 million has been raised through the Rita Hayworth Galas. These funds, combined with other donations, have helped the Alzheimer's Association make significant progress toward our mission to eliminate Alzheimer's disease.

Part the Cloud is committed to funding novel research ideas to determine if they will be effective treatments for the millions of people affected by Alzheimer's. While the vast increase in our understanding of Alzheimer's has led to the identification of promising targets for new therapies, the process of developing and testing potential therapies is long and complex, taking years and substantial resources. Many promising research ideas stall due to lack of funding. Most grants support middle and latter clinical trials, but there are few funding sources to support the earlier phase studies needed to test drug treatments in people. Part the Cloud addresses this critical gap, supporting early phase clinical studies and helping accelerate the transition of findings from the laboratory into possible therapies. Since 2012, Part the Cloud has generated more than $17 million in funding for Alzheimer's research, making it possible for the Alzheimer's Association to award 17 additional research grants during this time. These awards span a variety of targets in Alzheimer's disease research and fall under the leadership of some of the US's most prestigious scientists and universities.

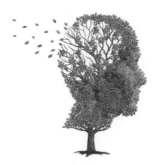

Battle tip: Raising awareness about dementia and its effects on individuals, their caregivers, and society is an important task for all of us. With rates of dementia growing, we, as a society, need to open the discussion about this problem.

Download Kit

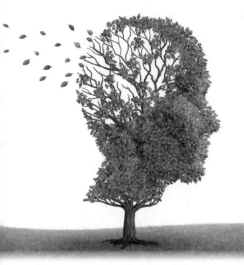

Please enter the URL you see in the box below in a web browser on your computer to access and use the download kit.

---

www.self-counsel.com/updates/dementiafamily/17kit.htm

The following files are included in the download kit:

- What to Ask When Choosing a Long-Term Care Facility
- What Might a Mini-Mental State Exam Be Like?
- Should You or a Loved One Visit a Doctor about Possible Dementia?
- Resources and Suggestions for Further Reading
- — And more!

OTHER TITLE OF INTEREST FROM SELF-COUNSEL PRESS

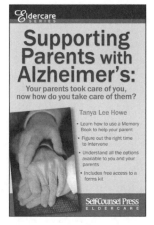

Supporting Parents with Alzheimer's:
You parents took care of you, now how do you take care of them?

Tanya Lee Howe

ISBN 978-1-77040-149-5

6 x 9 • paper + download • 144 pp.

First Edition

$19.95 USD/CAD

Many of us are unprepared and confused about how to proceed when a parent begins to suffer the effects of old age. This confusion is amplified when faced with the diagnosis of a cognitive illness such as Alzheimer's disease or other form of dementia. What can you do in the early stages? What if the illness has already progressed considerably but your parent still refuses your help? How do you give comfort?

Throughout the book, the author uses her own experiences to guide readers through the sensitive topic of eldercare. From deciding when to step in and help, how to care for your parent's emotional well-being, how to make health-care decisions, and how to help manage his or her finances, it explains it all.

If your parent has been diagnosed with a cognitive illness, *Supporting Parents with Alzheimer's* will arm you with the knowledge to meet your parent's psychological and physical needs so that he or she can continue to live comfortably and safely, without feeling like a burden.

The Author

Tanya Lee Howe is the author of *Start and Run a Tattoo & Body Piercing Studio*. Currently she is sharing care of a mother with Alzheimer's with her sister-in-law. They learned to communicate their day shift/night shift mother care by keeping a detailed journal.